How to Train Smart Even at Home

Functional Fitness Plan + Mental Training to Lose Weight

Larry Cole

ISBN Paperback: 978-1-80157-215-6

Printed by IngramSpark

First printing edition 2020.

Introduction

When you say the word health, you are referring to the wellbeing of yourself or others. So naturally, health becomes a personal matter especially when it revolves around your own health. Everyone wants to be in better health which is again a very natural impulse.

The first and easiest things you can do to better your health is to eat properly and work out routinely. Eating properly can be dieting and monitoring what comes into your kitchen. Working out, on the other hand, can be somewhat trickier.

Working out doesn't mean you have to

become a bodybuilder or weightlifter though those are possible achievements to gain from working out. It could simply mean you want to maintain a certain weight or keep your body moving properly and functionally. In such cases, to maintain proper health you don't need dumbbells and treadmills, only a functional fitness routine.

What is Functional Fitness?

Functional Fitness Defined

You may not have heard of the term functional fitness before reading this, but the truth is that functional fitness is all around you. Functional fitness refers to a type of fitness where you keep your body moving in simulated routines that resemble everyday tasks.

Now, most people imagine working out as this fantastical imagery where you have a solid core and large protruding biceps that bulge every time you lift weights. This image is one that's better to burn. Not everyone can live this fantasy and in most cases, it's unrealistic and impractical. It's more difficult to maintain a bulky, muscular physique than a normal one, and not many people are aiming to become a PRO bodybuilder.

An easier and more reasonable way to maintain a fit figure is by sticking to simpler goals. What most people want is to be able to perform with the most practicality on a daily basis. To ensure this, drop the weights and stick to more natural movements. This is where you'll resort to functional fitness.

With functional fitness, you'll be doing squats, lunges, stretches, and pumps that are closer to home. All of these movements will resemble the actions you do in everyday life.

Take lunges as an example. Lunges are the movement of stretching out and bending your leg. Though you'll never be found walking in this cycle, it's imitating the movements you make in more extreme cases. Going up the stairs and running use the same actions as walking does, but with more strength and power. By doing lunges, your muscles and joints become accustomed to the strong pull and strain and therefore perform more effectively as you run.

As you grow older, you may have found that your body can't do the same things as it used to. It's alright since this happens to everybody. Unfortunately, the more lethargic you become, the faster this will happen to you. So it's better to get up and get moving in any way that you can.

Functional Fitness can be performed anywhere at any level of difficulties. For instance, you can even use your own body weight to perform the exercises without using any gym equipment. As long as you're moving in a way that can benefit your body, you're doing some kind of functional fitness. It's better than lifting the heaviest weights and then snapping when you're trying to load groceries into your car.

Complimenting Functional Fitness with Your Lifestyle

As mentioned earlier, hoping for the perfect 10 out of 10 body is unrealistic and quite impractical. The basic aim should always be maintaining a healthy body you as a person are satisfied with.

Being fit is only an extra benefit to yourself. That said, your exercises shouldn't interrupt your schedule, but rather flow inside of it. Once it becomes a problem to find time for your workout, a red flag should signal in your mind. Here are some tips to keep in mind when crafting a workout routine that works for you.

Firstly, it shouldn't take long at all. A 15 to 25-minute routine is enough to make a difference, so long as you're implementing this workout every day. You don't need anything that hard, just simple repetitive movements to properly pump your muscles. Your short workout can be early in the morning or after your busy day.

Typically, it's better to work out before you start your day's work, otherwise doing anything at the end of the day will tire you out more than you'd usually be. You can also develop intense strain and pain if you remain idle for too long after a workout.

Another idea is to spread out your workouts through the week. On days you're working, work out for only 15 minutes and on weekends or holidays, work out for 20-25 minutes. This way you won't tire yourself out when you have other things to do. Any system that suits your schedule is fine, so long as you're getting the essential minimum of 15 minutes.

When you start out, keep all of your moves minimalistic. Nothing too extravagant that'll pull your muscles before you've even used them. No weights in the beginning. They will strain your muscles far too quickly. Once you're used to the burn from simpler workouts, you can apply small two or three pound weights. Never start out big, as it's unhealthy, unrealistic and impractical.

When you're working out, keep some water nearby and put on your sports gear. Always keep yourself hydrated when working out and stay safe at all times.

Have lots of free space around you with a clean, carpeted floor or purchase yourself a yoga mat for moves where you bend or lie down. The more spacious your environment is, the safer it is to execute your workout effectively without injuring yourself.

Is Functional Fitness Right For You?

In contrast to popular belief, any given fitness program might not be a good fit for separate individuals. Though society has now made it something very normal, you may not fit in with this group of people that can work themselves to the bone.

If you're baffled, bear through for there is an explanation. Yes, it's true that functional fitness basically tries to cover all generic movements, reinforce your stamina, strength, and range of motion yet still, what about those people who can perform daily tasks and nothing more?

Illnesses, weakness, age, and injury can prevent you from doing more than what you're currently capable of. Though you may feel you're ready for more, your body may not be. Remember before anything else, there's no need to push limits that shouldn't be pushed.

In typical cases, functional fitness can cover most people's necessities. Whether you're hunting for a better body or a more productive day, functional fitness reaps the benefits to aid you down that road. But for those with physical restraints and disabilities, there's no harm in realizing what you're not capable of doing.

If you're injured, then it's momentary unless the after effect is lifelong. A scrape or bruise will put you down for a few days. Broken bones will keep you grounded for a much longer period and in some severe cases, the rest of your life. If bodily functions are really something you wish to improve though, then there's no reason for you to carelessly carry yourself around, injuring your limbs.

Other momentary obstacles can be surgery, pregnancy, traveling or moving and other impactful events in life. There's no way you can keep up working out each and every day especially if you have other things on your agenda to attend to. Fret not if you miss a day, simply get back into the routine as soon as you can. The longer you wait, the harder it'll be to return to your former glory.

As you grow older, you'll become more limited to what you can do. Bone health and newly developed issues have to be taken into account before you attempt any kind of workout.

Some people are born with permanent issues that prevent them from working in certain positions. There are many situations you may find yourself in; being born with weaker bone strength could mean you're incapable of working yourself past a certain degree. Breathing or digestive issues can also hold you down from working out since these areas will be directly affected.

Benefits of Functional Fitness

There are multiple benefits to functional fitness that can easily become part of your daily routine. To convince you further of the powerful impact functional fitness can have on your life, here are some benefits that functional fitness can provide you with.

Easier Movement

The more you practice, the better you will be in any exercise movement. Remember those days as an infant when you were clambering onto the furniture trying to figure out how to walk? Of course not, since you were after all an infant, but it's a perfect example for this point.

As an infant, you'd have always fallen over, cried a little, and then returned to your attempts to get up and walk. The more you did it, the better you got at doing it since your body steadily adjusted to the actions. The same procedure occurs when you're working out. The more you repeat these actions, the more accustomed your body gets to them and the easier they become to perform.

Once your body is used to these movements, running, bending down, jumping and heaving will all become a lot easier. That's why making functional fitness a daily part of your routine is so important. If you lose the momentum of working out regularly, you'll also lose the stability and consistency of your movements, and you may even get sore much quicker than you might have before.

The best part about functional fitness is that you can start anywhere with it. There's no grand expectation to meet or deadlines to pay up monthly subscription fees, just your own personal-made goals and free time.

Functional fitness in its most basic to most intense form will always remain a low impact workout. It means beginners can commence at an easy pace without the exhausting themselves. On the other hand, those who already have it implemented in their schedule will easily be able to pick up their pace without leaving their comfort zone.

Once you've gotten down the pattern of your functional fitness routine and you have a clear idea of what you're capable of, keeping yourself fit will never be easier. Movements are always done best in a flow. Without a system to your movements, you'll end up fumbling and tumbling in everything you do.

Practice makes perfect and this applies to everything. The more you do something, the more progress you'll endure to succumb to the best of your ability. So, for the best performance each day with fast and steady movements, functional fitness is the best solution to making your body perfectly functional.

Stronger Support and Immune System

Though you may not realize it immediately, when you work out your body becomes stronger. It's more resistant to attacks upon it. Now when saying attack, this doesn't refer to life threatening events, only simple accidents that can harm your body.

Scratches and bruises will have less effect on your body if you work out on the daily. Instead of having a throbbing bruise on your knee for days on end, it may hurt for a few hours and then feel like an irritating itch.

You'll also be able to handle more impact on your muscles while you're on the move. If running and going up the stairs were an issue before, working out can help you make those issues disappear. Functional fitness is the best kind of workout for improving your daily functional movements, since this is the primary focal point in all the exercises.

With each workout, you'll also feel a surge of adrenaline run through your veins, which is a good thing. Adrenaline gives you extra power and more stamina. When you need it, adrenaline will be provided to you at a faster rate than if you didn't work out.

Along with the buildup of adrenaline, there's also the buildup of stamina. With this, you'll be able to perform for longer periods of time and do more than you can usually do. If heaving the groceries tired you out before, then after proper functional fitness you'll be hearing more than bags with ease in no time.

Every day will be so much easier to conquer when your body is stronger and sturdier. You'll also feel more energized and confident as you grow stronger. Functional fitness can help you increase your general health in everyday life.

Functional fitness can also open more doors for you. You can try new sports or hobbies that involve going out with clearer certainty. With a newer, fitter you there is more you can do, more options you can discover. Stamina and strength aren't things you can develop overnight, but once you have them all of your days will change for the better. Walking to your work will seem less of a hassle. Running in the evening will appear to be more fun than irritating.

Though you'll never be able to compete with the heavy bodybuilders out there by only doing functional fitness, you can reach fuller potential in more material events in life. You can get a lot more done when you are functionally fit throughout your day.

Look Better, Feel Better

One thing everyone's been taught since youth is to always feel good about yourself. Though you may not dwell too much on this idea, it's actually a life changing mentality that can differentiate an optimist and a pessimist. Thinking positively about yourself is the key to a happier life for anyone's situation. Before accepting anyone else, accept yourself for who you are.

If you can't do that, then make yourself the person you want to be and accept that. If you feel negatively about yourself, it'll be hard to see anyone else positively. Negativity is an awful quality to have but unfortunately, it is more contagious than positivity.

So if you walk around with a hunched back and a grumpy expression all day, it's highly likely you're dampening someone else's morning even if that wasn't your intention. Rather than being the party pooper, try being the life of the party. Make yourself a more confident and happier person by working on the most important part of your life; yourself.

Functional fitness isn't that time

demanding. All you need to do is honor 15 - 30 minutes of your time. Truth is, most people become self-conscious about their physique at some moment in their life. Maybe it had hit you in high school, your co-workers unintentionally made broad shoulders part of the uniform, or your in-laws pointed it out a little louder than they should've. In any case, the idea isn't to feel bad about yourself, but to feel motivated to do something about it.

With little pushes in the beginning, the results will start slipping into your jeans easier, show under your old sweaters and shirts and make your belts fall. Then, by that time you'll be able to work harder for stronger results that will truly dazzle your peers.

Though the steps to get there aren't small, they are possible and not hard to walk. Some great results from functional fitness are heightened strength in your joints and limbs, greater resistance against physical impacts and a better posture. That's right, with all the work you're inputting to your joints and limbs, your posture will be heavily impacted. A straighter back, a courageous lift underneath your chin and strong shoulders all come from 15 minutes of functional fitness every day. Isn't that something worth working for?

Functional Fitness and Other Exercises

Functional fitness is commonly mistaken for any ordinary exercise and implemented into most typical workout sessions without anyone even realizing what it is. The fact is there's a difference between functional fitness and other exercises. Though the line between them may not be fully distinguishable at the moment, that'll all be cleared with the following comparisons between functional fitness and other types of exercises you may be familiar with.

1 - Bodybuilding

Bodybuilding focuses less on functional strength and overall mobility. Instead, it emphasize more on mind-muscle connection, time under tension for muscle synthesis. No doubt about it,

bodybuilding-style programs are great for overall fitness, but it doesn't compliment all functional fitness has to offer.

There are similarities between the two types of workouts. They both do help make for a better, stronger, healthier physical appearance, though one exaggerates it more than the other. A fit appealing body is what you'll get, but when it comes to similarities, that's all there is. Sometimes you may find some functional fitness moves in your bodybuilding workout but you'll never find primarily bodybuilding moves in a functional fitness routine.

Functional fitness focuses less on grinding your muscles and more on your flexibility and higher standard strength in tasks you'll encounter. When it comes to the daily routine, functional fitness is the helping hand holding you steady while you work through the day.

When you're a bodybuilder, being the handy average Joe isn't what you're aiming for. Instead, it's more like you're aiming to be the extraordinary model people look up to and gaze appreciatively towards. Bodybuilders are built to appear tough, but the truth is that they're not that tough.

When working on your muscles the bodybuilder way, the only thing you're doing is heightening the pulse and intensity of your muscles. Some core muscles in your limbs are completely skipped over and therefore not as strong as they could be. So while a bodybuilder has the look, they might not have the strength their muscles falsely portray.

Bodybuilders are actually pretty delicate. They can't take hardy impacts with swollen muscles and may have a harder time carrying themselves if they don't properly use their newfound power. When you're working out on a daily basis with the aim of greater performance in chores, you'll achieve that goal. When you work to make the perfect vision, then by all means you'll get what you want but then it's up to you to carry that proud physique.

2 - Heavy Weight Training

This is no stranger to most people's vocabulary. We've all seen how the strongmen in society lift the heaviest of weights with ease and blow our minds away. This is an extraordinary act indeed, but when will you ever do something that out of the ordinary in your daily life?

Functional fitness is quite similar to weightlifting and bodybuilding in various ways. You'll get the body and appearance you want and most likely more than those of a normal functional fitness routine. You'll also be able to lift amazingly heavy weights which is great, right? Not in every case.

In the gym it might be a bragging right, or when you're starting a conversation about your hard core hobbies. When it comes to working at home though, lifting a box off the floor might strain your back painfully, even if it's a light box.

As mentioned earlier, functional fitness works on your daily life, making tasks you do each day easier and less of a hassle to perform. Steadily, each chore becomes easier as you get better. Functional fitness figuratively lightens the weights on your shoulders that were placed there.

Weight lifters can easily lift weights off

of their shoulders, but only when they are in the proper position, with enough strength and utilizing the right equipment. Those who weightlift obviously know that there are protocols and conditions to be met when becoming weightlifters. How to prop yourself with the equipment, how to hold the bar of the dumbbell, and how to keep posture when holding the weights airborne. These are all things you prepare to do when weightlifting.

An easier way to think of it is so; when becoming a weightlifter, you are preparing for the next meet, achieving the next Personal Best. When you're focusing on functional fitness, you're focusing more on preparing yourself for better health, mobility and the ability to handle daily activities with ease. So when it comes to practicality, functional fitness carries more weight.

Functional fitness targets if not all then most of the muscles you use on a daily basis. By gradually strengthening them through a series of exercises, they become more efficient and perform to higher degree. When weightlifting, you only focus on strengthening those muscles that will help you lift the heavy weights. This is fine as long as you are only planning on using those muscles for heavy lifting.

The primary issue when it comes to weightlifting is the way you're doing it. You're either propped in a seated position or lying down, a steady pose that isn't going to harm the rest of your body. After weightlifting for quite some time, weightlifters' muscles will become accustomed to this same pattern of movement in order to be more efficient with their lifts. However, when it comes to any other unconventional exercises out of their usual lifting patterns (such as Bench Press, Squats and Deadlifts), they often struggle.

3 - Group Training

When you're training by yourself in your own home, you have the luxury of comfort and solitude. Anything you're doing suits your needs. All you have to do is make an environment that's fit for fitness and you're well on your way towards a healthy lifestyle. The making of your new person is done by your hand, which is pressure on no one else but yourself.

What about when you work in a group? In a group you have an instructor, which is a hefty pro since they know what they're doing and teaching. When you're working with a professional instructor, there's a greater environment of motivation to endure the workouts for a better appearance and healthier body. Those people around you could be friends or at least acquaintances that want to achieve the same goal as you, making a friendly environment.

The environment itself is one carefully designed to cater the needs of a workout. So you have the proper space, the proper colleagues and the proper instructor. It sounds great so far.

Now here's where the hill drops. When you're working in a group, the catering isn't personal and generalized so that it fits a popular demand. Your demand may not be popular and you may find difficulty keeping up with the crowd. If you have a disability or any type of illness that prevents you from performing certain actions, you may as well not be a part of the group.

When you're working by yourself the workout can be adapted to suit all of your own needs and run to your own pace rather than the pace of others and an instructor who is already fit as a fiddle. So keep in mind all the time what it is you're looking for from your workouts to decisively decide what it is you need and remember, functional fitness is a category of its own.

Common Mistakes with Functional Fitness

Functional fitness is a great way to get yourself into shape, as long as you're doing it right. If you're confused, then the easiest way to word it is, you can work out wrong.

There are many common mistakes most people make when they start working out by themselves or even when they're starting out in a gym. So, before you start out on your own routine, make sure to do some research and learn the correct forms of execution.

An Everyday Routine

One mistake people tend to make all too often is doing the same workout every single day. If you do this, you'll never get the ideal muscles, tone, and body that you want. Yes, over time these workout sessions will get easier and you'll feel the strength in your limbs while doing this, but watch yourself crumble when you have to try a different workout.

Your body is made up of many limbs,

muscles, bones and joints. If you don't work on all of these parts of your body equally, you'll end up with an imbalance in your strength and stamina which results in nothing good.

Any good workout will have multiple actions that'll target specific muscles in your body. When you combine the four main components of fitness (discussed in later chapters) you get the right balance between everything your body needs.

Unfortunately this isn't as easy as piecing a puzzle together. Instead, it's more like having to make smaller puzzles first in order to make a larger one. Once one component has been completed, you move on to the next one. This is a timely process which can't all be tackled in one workout.

So when one workout focuses on cardio and perhaps muscle building, another workout you do through the week can focus more on HIIT and stretching. Keep switching up your exercises rather than doing the same one each day. Take it slow, only change your routine when you know you can handle new moves and challenges.

If you constantly swap your daily exercise, you'll cover more ground quicker and spread the oncoming strength to all parts of your body. Only doing one type of exercise is going to tire you out and not properly help your body develop the way you'd have wanted it to.

Love What You Do

Some people work out because they feel they have to with no other choice. No one can truly determine your own situation quite like you can, but this is the wrong mentality. You should never approach your workout sessions with resentment. Always look to your workouts with optimism and confidence.

If you want to work out, then do it for yourself, not for anyone else's satisfaction. If you feel that you're being pressured into working out then the results are never going to satisfy you, even if you do make it to your goal.

You have to enjoy something in order to achieve anything. If you don't like cooking, then you'll never enjoy a meal even if you mastered the recipe. The victory is always sweeter when you've got sugar, not salt.

Start working out when you feel good about working out. Do workouts that make you feel confident you have what it takes to make the change you need. If you don't like the criticism, comparisons or judgement of others, then don't go to the gym. You don't need to be in a crowd to get the motivation you need to starting lifting weights and running in evenings.

All your motivation should be positive, not negative. When you have positive motivation, it means you are being forward by the achievement you'll receive. When you have negative motivation, it means you are driven by the consequences of not acting. Don't be afraid of what people are going to say and do if you don't work out, think about all of the good response you'll get from doing so. Remember how happy you'll be when you finally reach where you want to be. Keep all of your thoughts positive and you'll not only feel good, but soon enough you'll look good as well.

Dieting

Another one of the most common

mistakes people make when they're starting out, they think they have to start dieting! No matter what science and TV health programs try to tell you, dieting isn't the perfect solution for weight issues. Nowadays, people are coming to realize that diets actually limit you way too much.

When you start dieting, you work with either elimination or restriction. This should never be the case. Eat as much as you can permit yourself to. Have a balance of everything edible out there. Nothing should stop you from eating what you wish.

Just have a balance with what you eat.

Most of your normal diet should consist of healthy hearty foods and whatever little snack your gluttony craves for can be satisfied once in a while. There is no issue with having a treat after some time. Keep control over how much junk food you have and keep that careful eye over your food to make sure the good always outweigh the bad.

Working out doesn't make dieting compulsory. If anything, it means you have to keep yourself energized more often. You'll crave more food once you start working out and that craving is one you're going to want to satisfy. If not, you'll become grumpy, hungry and your attitude towards working out won't be a very positive one.

Rolling with No Goals

There's no race to be won if there's no finish line. You always have to chart out your goals before you start working on a project.

In this case, the project is yourself, and you need to place some goals on what you want to do. Do you eventually want to have that hard core six pack? Are you aiming for a fitter, stronger you? Lay out your goal and make it clear to yourself, otherwise you may as well be running head first into fog.

Once believe you have a goal, set down your stepping stones to get there. You can't just hope you can make the jump from your side to the finish line. Make the bridge and cross it one tile at a time. It's a timely process, but it'll grant you the guaranteed success you want. It's better to work your way through at a decent pace rather than failing and having to restart the whole process.

First, try to lose weight. Aim for something that's fit and healthy. Go for at least 10 pounds less than what you are now. By the time you've reached that goal, you'll have gotten accustomed to the fatigue and strain after a hefty workout session. You'll also have a stronger understanding of how much you can handle and where the limit can't be breached.

Then, try aiming for another goal. Seek to tone your muscles a little bit at first, so you can understand how much time it takes you. Once you've gotten a clearer idea, you can start working hard to the final destination.

All of this will take a decent amount of time so don't give up if the results don't show after weeks, or maybe even a month. They'll come along soon and once they do it'll have been worth all of the time and effort.

The First Component of Functional Fitness: Power

When you first think of the word power, you may think of the word strength next. When it comes to working out though, this isn't the case. Power and strength are two different aspects when it comes to exercise, each targeting and influencing different parts of the body.

What is Power?

Power refers to your speed in doing something. When you're performing an act at high speed and fluency, such as jumping and running, this is referred to as your power.

Power does have other meaning in other situations, such as the power or influence you have over someone or a certain situation, but this does not apply to exercise.

When you say that somebody is powerful in terms of their physique, you refer to the speed it takes someone to do something. To clarify this point, consider the following example.

When you're capable of doing 50 push ups continuously, you're considered strong because of this capability. If you can do 50 push ups in two minutes, you'd be considered strong. But if the person next to you can do 50 push ups in half that time, they would be considered more powerful than you.

The same applies even when you're competing in sports. In swimming, if you and another person can only do 5 laps in one go, you're both as strong as each other. But if the person swimming alongside you can do it in seven minutes while you do it in ten, they're more powerful than you.

You can have the same level of strength as someone, but not the same level of power. Having the same amount of strength as someone isn't that hard to achieve as you may think. When it comes to having the same amount of power though, it becomes very challenging to find someone on the exact same level as you.

Don't get the wrong idea though, power and strength are both connected. Power actually is a combination of speed and the strength you have in order to do something. Without adequate strength, you won't have any power to exert.

You'll also find that over a period of time, you'll lose your power faster than you lose your strength. This is because overtime your body adjusts to wielding the strength it has, but as your body's original shape deteriorates over the years, your joints and muscles don't react as quickly as they would've done before.

Power is much harder to maintain than your level of power. The most common way to enhance your power would be by applying heavier weights to your workout so that you can perform your actions with greater resistance.

To further understand why you need to maintain your level of power, think of all the places where you need to be quicker and have more speed.

Power in your Daily Life

You can develop greater power to enhance your strength and speed. With all things you do, there's a certain amount of strength and ability required. Moving around items in your house requires strength you may not use on a daily basis. Cleaning for example, sweeping and dusting depend on a consistent movement of swaying your arm to and fro. You can have this strength to do to continuously, but do you have the power to do it quickly enough.

With power comes more valuable time in your grasp. How so? Think of all the things you have to do in one day. There are some things that will inevitably take time, like driving during traffic, waiting on the elevator and holding your spot in line during rush hour at the cafe. But during the day, there are things you can control such as climbing the stairs, walking or even getting ready in the morning.

If you can better the actions you have control over every day, you can spare yourself more time and energy for those things beyond your control. With more time you'll also have more stamina for the rest of your day. Some people are pooped after their daily morning routine and if that's you, then there's no way you're getting through the day on an energized positive principle.

You shouldn't be crawling on all fours to get through your day, you should be walking with stride each day, invigorated and prepared for the following days.

This is why you need power throughout your day. You don't have to be a strongman to have power. Any ordinary person can enhance their power to become a better more efficient version of themselves. Through progressive workouts you can improve your performance.

Think of power as the applications on a device to ease your understanding. Your phone would be your strength. With your phone you're able to call people anywhere you go. With applications, you can do more at faster speeds. You have access to social media and games. The more applications you have, the more you can do in less time. With only a phone, you have a base. With applications, you build up on that base to make it stronger.

Power Moves

A note to remember; when it comes to most exercise moves, they've already combined all four components of functional fitness into the exercise. The following exercises are examples of those that you can use to gain benefit in all fields including power, with these reasons further explained.

1. Jump squats

Jump squats are great for enhancing your core and leg power. This gives you the strength to withstand the resistance of squatting or simply bending down. With this move, you can bend your knees easier, knees being a primary area that wear out the fastest.

You don't have to jump in this move if it's your first time. You can simply squat to alleviate the strain off this motion.

2. Dumbbell Curl

This move is by far the easiest to introduce to your workout. Take one dumbbell in each hand and curl your arms at a steady pace. This helps you improve your general arm strength.

With this, your arms won't succumb to heavy burdens when you pick up larger objects. The dumbbell curl can be made harder by holding your positions longer, introducing squats alongside the move or by lifting the dumbbells over your head and then dropping them before curling your arms. Of course all of these moves should be done after you're properly accustomed to regular dumbbell curves.

3. Plyo Lateral Lunge

Rather than the usual lunge facing forward, take your lunges to the side. Stand straight with your arms down and move your left leg outward to the left. Stretch your left leg out so that it is straight, but your right leg is bent and go as far down as you comfortably can.

This will help your legs adapt to a side movement and strain from the upper body. This can help with extending your leg and bending down. When you feel comfortable with this move, introduce weights or resistance bands under your straightened leg. This will help the buildup strength in your legs.

4.   Burpee

This move is both as classic as it is functional. Your entire body's accustomed to general strain, from crouching to bending down to jumping all in one fluent move.

Start by going down with your knees bent to your chest and then pump them out so you're in a planking position. After doing this, bring your legs back to your chest and jump upwards. As soon as you land flat on your feet, repeat this cycle.

To make this slightly more challenging, bring your knees up to your chest while you're jumping. That way your jumps have a stronger spring to them.

The Second Component of Functional Fitness: Strength

Next on the list of components is the mighty force of strength. Strength is what most people tend to pay attention to, though it isn't the only thing that makes you a stronger person as a whole. Strength is the foundation you want to be sturdy and reliable in order for you to build over it.

What is Strength?

Strength has been mentioned in the previous chapter quite a bit, but never properly defined. Strength, when it comes to fitness, is defined as exerting force against some kind of resistance.

Everyone has their own level of strength; In your daily life, if you pay close attention to all you do, you'll come to realize that there are many times when you apply strength.

You'll also notice that not all strength is the same. There are different types of strength that you apply every day, those being;

1. **Maximum Strength.** This is the most amount of strength you can possibly exert in one go. Rolling your sleigh down the slide, you'll want to use your maximum strength to get the best push down for more fun. It's all you can do in the moment and if you have great strength levels, that's a lot of fun down the hillside.

2. **Elastic Strength.** This one needs slightly more explanation. Think of an elastic band and how fast it reacts when you let it go. It reacts similar to a whiplash, for a fast and extremely hardy impact. When you have elastic strength it means you're capable of reacting to resistance with a fast or

elastic contraction.

3. **Strength Endurance.** This is the ability to repeat an action over and over at the same consistency. Think of a baseball player, mainly looking at the pitcher. Every time they throw the ball, they're expected to throw it at the same speed and force as the last time they did before. This is where you'll note their strength endurance.

All these types of strength have their own focused exercises that help enhance your durability in these fields. Without these strengths, there'd be a lot you wouldn't be able to do. They can all also be specialized in. So if you only work on your strength and endurance, you may not have optimum elastic strength.

When it comes to all strength training, you focus on the muscles connected directly to your bones. These are the muscles that work directly with your movements and therefore have greater impact on how strong the outcome of your movement is.

Strength training is often the first item on any workout list since it's the foundation of all physical ability. When you have a sturdy enough base, you can move on to other focal exercises that centre other objectives to be dealt with.

If strength training isn't what you primarily targeted, then you may encounter issues with other workouts that turn out to be specialized in focusing on other functional aspects.

Strength in your Daily Life

You don't have to go to the gym to be strong.

Strength applies to all aspects of our life. You can be emotionally strong, mentally strong, socially strong and more. In this case, you're concentrating on your physical strength. Physical strength is used in every move you make. When you walk, run, jump, heave and shove, you're using your strength to do so.

When heaving large boxes, you'll be using your maximum strength when picking one up. After that, it's maintenance of your strength level to carry the box to where it needs to be. If you do this action over and over again, you'll be using your strength endurance to withstand the constant strain created by the additional weights.

If for instance, the box slips from your hands while you're walking, you'd use your elastic strength to stabilize your grip. As soon as your box starts slipping, your reaction timing and elastic strength would work together to make sure you don't completely drop the box.

All of your strengths work together every day to make sure you're always ready to take the load of the day.

Another thing to note is that not all strength is trained with weights, but mainly resistance. Making the break between your exercises and repeating actions intensely are great ways to enhance your performance. Core workouts and complex sessions with greater variety all cover the muscles you need to bulk when working out.

Strength workouts should never be intense when you're starting out. They should be easy low level workouts with minimal variety. Your body needs to accustom to the new impact the workout is going to leave on you. You might have to take a break for the next 1 or 2 days if you're starting anew.

Strength Moves

Strength exercise should always target your entire body. Since strength has to be your foundation for all of your physical activities, it's better if you get all the body parts pumped and ready for action in one go.

Most exercise moves that emphasize strength will recommend the use of weights. So when it comes to creating a heavily strength exercise routine, weights, resistance bands and yoga balls are your key to finding the right way to truly test your limits.

1. Single Leg Bridge

In this move, you'll be coordinating your leg and core for dual coverage. Lying face up, lift your leg until it's at a 45 degrees into the air. Then lift your stomach a little to raise your leg higher. This move should be done as a pump, so that there's more burn with each repetition.

This move helps coordinate the core with the legs, resisting strain and pressure. You can implement this move with a crunch or with leg weights to make it more intense.

2.   Split Squat

With this squat, you make it harder for yourself, creating more strain and resistance. For this move you're not going to need weights, but a chair. Placing the chair behind you, place your foot on it so that one leg is bent and the other is straight. Then, step forward and squat with the leg not on the chair.

Do this with the other leg, swapping them to and fro until you feel the intense burn.

This means the workout is working and you're developing better leg strength.

3.   Glute Bridge

With this move, what you'll be doing is lying down on your back, and lifting your glute only in a pump movement. This will strengthen your core as a whole whenever you're going to bend or stretch your stomach.

You can place weights in your hands while lifting your stomach, lifting the weights to increase both your arm and core strength.

4.   Bent-Knee Calf Raise

For this workout you're going to need a box to step over. Stand straight on your box, arms straight down and legs spread shoulder width apart. Have a weight in each hand while they hang. Lift one of your legs up and have your other leg bent slightly on the box. Focus on concentric and eccentric movement of your calves while doing this for sets of 15-20 reps. Do this on each leg one after the other for greater effect.

The Third Component of Functional Fitness: Range of Motion

Next along the list of what contributes to your functional fitness workout is your range of motion. Your range of motion is defined as the measurement of movement around a specific body part.

What is Range of Motion?

Think of how far you can stretch your leg over the stairs. You might be able to stretch your leg to the second step, you might make it to the third. If you're tall enough, stretch all the way to the fourth but keep in mind, you're using your range of motion as you're doing this.

Range of motion can be associated with your flexibility, but they aren't entirely the same thing. Flexibility is the abstract movements your body can perform. Range of motion is quite literally the range of how far you can go. So when you work on your flexibility, you're also working on extending your range of motion.

Your range of motion is what allows to extend your reach and keep your limbs alive, ready and always moving. Your range of motion relates to how well you can move around, how far your reach can go. Being strong is great, but if you can't reach the top shelf without stretching a muscle, then you're missing out on a few vital exercises.

Range of motion mainly comes from stretches. You should occasionally stretch your limbs in all directions where you can comfortably go. This way, you keep a hold of your range of motion. Range of motion is as easy to lose as your power is. Once you've lost the flow or routine of strengthening it, it's really hard to get it back.

Range of motion may not seem that important on its own but combined with the other components of functional fitness it really makes the difference between one person and another. You may have immense power and strength, but without a decisive range of motion, you'll never be the best runner since your legs aren't accustomed to taking such large steps.

With power and strength, you can run consistently at a fast pace, which is good. To make yourself better, you'd improve the length of your stride by stretching your legs during exercises.

Never think of the components of functional fitness as isolation movements as they require multiple muscles synergy to perform each exercise. When they work together, they create a strong, sturdy base that you can rely on every single day.

Range of Motion in your Daily Life

Range of motion applies to everything you do, though you may not notice it in your daily actions. When you stretch to reach something overhead, when you take a longer stride to step over a puddle, when you kneel down to find something hidden under your bed, they're all examples of range of motion in your life.

When you work on your range of motion, you not only work on extending your reach, but also on making it easier for you to reach that far.

Think of the athletic performance that you can bring over to daily activities. It'll be easier to run, jump and walk at a faster pace. You can stretch overhead and below yourself effortlessly. Actions in general become much easier.

When you work out, you do actions in a more exaggerated manner than what they really are in real life. This technique ensures that anything you do in your daily routines remains something easily doable.

Range of motion isn't something you work on, on its own. It's interpreted with everything you do in real life and in your workout session. Though you'll find workouts that convey they are primarily range of motion workouts, they'll actually have a secondary focal point that additionally trains your range of motion.

The best part about training your range of motion is that it can be as easy as stretching in the morning. After you wake up, roll over to the side of the bed and stretch your arms over your head. Rattle your legs a little bit and arch your back. All of these can help day by day to make your reach a little better than it was yesterday.

Have a yoga session. Go out for a run. Doing the smallest of things can help your range of motion. The more you do it, the greater its development. So as long as you endlessly keep at it every day for even 15 minutes, you'll feel and see the difference.

Range of Motion Moves

These actions are better done in between at the beginning and in the end of your workout. All of these moves are done better when you hold them for minimum 20 seconds each.

1. Lunge with a Spinal Twist

It's the usual lunge with a new twist for you to try out. Once you're in the lunge stance, place one hand down on the floor and the other in the air, twisting your core so that you're facing upwards. Turn between your arms, taking your movements slowly.

This helps your core, leg and arm stretch. All is done in one move and the longer you hold it, the stronger the burn and the easier it'll be the next time you do it.

2.   Butterfly Stretch

Rather than stretching your limbs outwards, bring them all inwards so that you're comfortable in closed positions. Sit down and bring your feet together, making them touch each other's soles. Place your right hand on your left shin and left hand on right shin.

Keep this pose for as long as you can, standard 20 seconds to have best effect.

3.   Seated Shoulder Squeeze

In this move, you're sitting on the floor quite like how you did in the Butterfly Stretch, only this time you take your arms to your back and clasp them together.

Immediately you should feel your shoulder bones constraining in the pose.

The Fourth Component of Functional Fitness: Balance and Endurance

Finally, to complete the set of four, there's the last and final component, balance and endurance. These two work together in all ways and help enhance everything you can do, including the other components listed above.

What is Balance and Endurance?

Balance and endurance both have separate definitions. Balance is defined as your capability to control, handle and manage your body's movement. There are two types of balance to consider, those being your static balance and your dynamic balance. Static balance refers to the balance you must acquire while you're stagnant, completely still. This type of balance is easier to learn to control

over your dynamic balance which is your level of balance when you're mobile.

An addition to balance would be coordination, which is a very important theory in fitness. Coordination is the capability to do two or more things at once, move your body in two or more different ways with fluency and efficiency.

Balance and coordination go hand in hand, and held in your other hand would be endurance. Endurance, which can also be referred to as stamina, is the ability of your muscles and body to remain active during a lengthy period of time.

Together, balance and endurance help create a set time limit of how long you can do something. With good balance and standard endurance, you'll be active for a long amount of time.

This leads to the final summary of all the components of functional fitness. With the proper amount of strength, you have a solid base to becoming a fit person. Your strength is going to help you withstand all the restraint you'll experience while you're working out.

Power is the speed that you can apply to your workouts to handle them quicker and with more force. Power helps build up your strength so that there's more to exert, helping you reach the extra mile.

The other way you're going to reach the extra mile is by using your range of motion, which is going to help reach further in a shorter amount of time. Don't get power and range of motion confused. Power will take you faster, range of motion will take you further. Together they create a useful duo.

Finally there's your balance and endurance. They're the components that give you a time limit on how long you can last at peak performance. There's a limit to everything and eventually you'll wear down. Your balance will falter and your breaths harsher and raspier.

Put them all together and you have all of the pieces to create the perfect complete puzzle to understanding your maximized personal health.

Balance and Endurance in your Daily Life

Balance and endurance keep you running through the day in the most minimal way. They go together as well as rhymes do, harmoniously ensuring that you have the equity and stamina to progress through the events occurring all day. As the saying goes, everything works when there's a balance.

The simplest and most relatable example would have to be when going up the stairs. While going up the stairs, each moment you lift your foot is a split second of momentary balance. Without that balance, you'd go tumbling down the stairs.

In this case, you'd also require the stamina to keep going up flights of stairs. With the right amount of stamina, you can make it up the entire staircase, but without it you'll be wheezing after the third flight.

Balance and endurance are actually two things you can't notice quite easily. These two attributes keep improving on a daily basis, and contracting at the same time. The more you do in one day, the better you'll be tomorrow. The less you do today, the less you'll be able to do tomorrow.

If you consistently improve your balance and endurance, you'll consistently get better results. But balance, coordination and endurance aren't aspects you can simply stop working on. As soon as you find yourself on a suitable level of endurance, you keep at it.

Maintain your level and never fall from it. As you get older, it'll be harder to keep one level so it's better to maintain rather than trying to climb any higher. Just as well, if you stop working on them, your balance and endurance are going to fall by the day.

Cleaning, cooking, walking, talking these are all things that take up your endurance. Running, heaving, any sort of movement with any part of your body all require some balancing effort.

Without proper care, walking will become a chore and you'll become lethargic without the right level of stamina.

Balance and Endurance Moves

You can have a full yoga session once or twice a week to cover this type of workout.

1. One Leg Stand

With this workout, you'll be standing with one leg airborne and the other one rooted to the floor. Try holding this pose for as long as you can.

At first you might want to hold on to a wall or chair so you can better adjust to the pose. If your balance is generally not good, then start with your arms stretched outwards for greater balance.

If you have better balance, then complicate this easy step by pumping your elevated leg. This way you can better both your balance and your power with one move.

2. Plyo Lunge

In this version of a lunge, every time you bend down over one leg, you're going to jump and swap to the other leg. In this manner you're going to help enhance your endurance with each swap, imitating the actions you do when running.

Plyo lunge is a more intense move than a normal lunge so please don't try it unless you're comfortable and more than capable of doing a regular lunge first.

3. Straight-leg Calf Raise

With this move, your balance will be intensely tested. Standing on a step or box with your heels hanging over the edge, lift one leg behind yourself. Push your foot up so that you're on your toes, hold for a few seconds and then come back down. Swap your legs after a few pumps on each foot.

This is going to hurt when you do it, but you'll surely have better balance after this.

The Power of Mind in Weight Loss

We will begin this journey of reforming our perceptions about weight loss by going back to all we know about losing weight. We will focus on the concept most loss weight programs revolve around. Know that we are not just going to learn about these concepts but look to affirm its authenticity in losing weight. We have read stories and even experience not losing weight even after going on a supposed "quick weight loss diet." There are countless fad diets out there, and we need to learn the basics of staying fit rather than letting the opinions of dietitians influence our perceptions. No, I am not going to share my ideas or opinions because I will also fall into that category. What we will learn is facts and not suggested-truths.

Weight Loss and Fat Loss

Losing weight and burning fat is a bit different. However, fat loss is a subset of weight loss. But do you know that what most of us do is lose fat? Sometimes, we use the phrases interjectively without knowing which is which.

So, you want to lose weight? But is that what you mean? Weight loss is the decrease in our overall body weight. You don't just lose the body fat hanging around your triceps, belly, and thigh; you lose muscles and water in your body.

Muscle loss

Muscle loss happens when you build a weight loss program around reduced-calorie. This is entirely absurd, but reducing your calorie consumption shouldn't be your only objective. This will result in weight loss, primarily in loss of muscle tissue. Hence, you might not lose as much fat as you would want;

instead, you shred your muscles. You lose more tissue weight when you engage in an intensive cardio workout while you reduce your calorie intake. This happens because your body needs the macronutrient unavailable due to calorie restrictions to build up those muscles while you work out.

Know that one pound of muscle weight lost equals a pound of fat. This means if you lose 10 pounds of fat, it's the same as losing 10 pounds of muscle tissue. Regardless the latter is denser and harder. When you lose muscle weight, you might notice your body change, but not necessarily in the area, you want. Well, body fat is a bit more obvious than muscle tissues.

Water loss

Calorie restriction and cardio workouts cause muscle loss while focusing on cutting carbs results in water weight. This is because carbohydrate retains more water, 3 times actually than other macronutrients such as protein. So, when you reduce how much carbs you consume, your body isn't retaining as much water as usual. In a few weeks on a low carb diet, your muscles adapt to dehydration and begin to shrink, causing water loss in the body.

On the other hand, fat loss is shredding your body fat situated in your face, neck, belly, triceps, and thigh region. Wondering how you still count-off some pounds after weeks of being on a diet? Well, whether you focus on losing weight or just body fat, it causes a decrease in your overall weight. The only difference is that with weight loss, you lose more pounds compared to fat loss.

I need you to get from all this because your overall weight is not a statement of how fat you are. At 25, you might think that weighing 130lbs shows you are fat even when there is no physical testament to that and feel the need to lose weight to feel secure. You are not fat; you have more muscles built. You can *incorporate different dietary plans adapting to your preferences. Knowing the difference between weight loss and fat loss will help you recognize which is best for your body. Thus, you are on the path to a successful weight/fat loss journey.*

Calories Vs. Carbs

Should you focus on cutting calories or carbohydrates?

The different diet suggests one or the other towards the same result: weight loss. People get confused as to which is the best for them. This confusion is entirely down to the many disadvantages of sugar. Sugary foods and carbohydrates go together. For instance, the Low-Carb Diet advises that we reduce our consumption of carbs to lose weight. On the other hand, the Standard diet pushes us towards cutting calories. So, to reduce your weight, should you cut your sugar-based foods intake or reduce your calorie consumption?

Naturally, you must cut your calories towards weight loss because your body needs to burn more than you consume. That way, you lose weight and not gain more in the process of that. Imagine someone spending an hour on a treadmill and going ahead to order 2 cheeseburgers from McDonald's. This individual just wasted an hour on the treadmill. So, calorie restriction is an important part of your weight loss journey or a plan to lose only body fat.

Carbohydrates, on the other hand, accounts for four calories per gram compared to 9 calories per gram of fat. This shows that you should actually look to cut bad fat from your diet compared to carbohydrates; excluding refined carbs, as these are a no, no.

I used the phrase "bad fat/cholesterol" because we also have good ones. Low-Density Lipoprotein, LDL, is regarded as bad cholesterol as high-level build-up cholesterol which clogs the arteries, which prompts health conditions such as obesity, heart disease, and stroke. High-Density

Lipoproteins, HDL, are the good guys designed to counter the progress of LDL.

When it comes to weight loss, both carbs and calorie count apply. Although few diet plans will argue with this, you will need to watch both your calories and carbohydrates intake for a healthier you while losing weight.

It would be best if you had a balance of fat, carbs, and protein, whether you look to lose weight or not. This ensures you don't fall into any health complications while you attempt to lose weight. So, count your calories, at the same time, ensure you keep to a balanced meal. With enough nutrients (scattered in all kinds of food), your body functions appropriately, keeping it healthy.

To know the number of calories you need to consume, you have to first find out your Base Mass Index, BMI (weight in km/height in m2). With your BMI, you could use a fitness tracker to know the number of calories you need to consume each day. Knowing our body calorie capacity helps us to eat how much our body needs in a day. Going beyond that leads to weight gain as the body looks to process and store those extra calories.

Dieting Myths

When it comes to weight-loss diets, there are lay down rules you have to follow. Adhering to these regulations is vital to losing weight healthily. However, this mentality has opened a weight loss diet to some myths. Unfortunately, hundreds of individuals are convinced by these mistakes. It is vital that in your weight loss journey, you can separate them from facts. This will inarguably make the journey worthwhile. You don't have to worry about why you might not be shredding those pounds. With that, let some prevalent diet myths that you should be wary of.

Skipping meals will help lose weight faster

This idea is very popular. Most people will tell you it works. The truth is it works a bit only for about a few weeks, and then you gain those weights again. On the other hand, dietitians do not advise you to skip meals. Do you know why? Not eating breakfast, lunch, or dinner makes your weight loss journey difficult. Naturally, adopting a diet to lose weight is challenging. However, if you decide to resist taking a lunchbox to work, you only just made it more challenging to keep up with your new diet. Skipping meals leads to cravings, and these also prompt you to make unhealthy decisions. You are more likely to reach for that favorite and heavily sweetened drink of yours when you fail to eat.

Staying away from treats

Staying away from those treats is yet another weight loss idea people get wrong. Yes, those threats are likely to dampen the outcome. However, this happens only when you eat a lot of them. Diet plans do not necessarily have to cue in a stringent lifestyle. There are rules, but these guidelines are often taken too far. You can indulge yourself in a treat every once in a while. What you do is curb what you eat. When you stay away from your favorite foods that are loaded with unhealthy fats, you will eventually give in. When this happens, you will want to make up for lost times by consuming in excess. Consequently, you add more weight than you lose.

You can't eat late at night
Almost every diet plan constitutes this myth, or at least what people say it is. The conclusion is that when you eat late, your body is unable to digest the food. A slow metabolism makes it difficult to lose weight. There is, without a doubt, that late-night eating before bed leads to indigestion and, most likely, heartburn. Nevertheless, this happens when you consume a large portion— nibbling on a healthy snack before bed will not disrupt your weight loss diet.

Stay away from fatty foods

Foods high in fat are good at the same time bad for us. How? There are two kinds of fat: healthy and unhealthy fats. Eating either of these impacts your cholesterol levels: High-density Lipoprotein, HDL, and Low-density Lipoprotein, LDL. LDL is responsible for the accumulation of body fat in the form of a plague. HDL, on the other hand, helps remove these fats through your liver.

Now, eating foods high in unhealthy fat, such as saturated fat, raises both cholesterol levels. However, you need HDL to increase, not LDL. This is where healthy fats such as monounsaturated fats help clean off LDL. See, some fatty foods lead to weight loss. Examples of foods with healthy fat include avocados, cheese, and dark chocolate.

Note that there aren't specific foods that help burn fat; it all boils down to balancing your diet.

Carbs are the source of your body fat

Now, this is another mistake that has a huge followers' base. Carbohydrate dense foods contain fat but not as much as you think. It is all about choosing the right carbs to eat and curbing your food portion when you do so. You don't necessarily have to keep clear of them to avoid weight gain. Watch out for foods that are high in calories, especially the ones that need toppings or fillings like pasta. These will increase the amount of fat you consume. Regardless, carbs are not fattening when you control your portions at the same time being selective of them. Go for whole grains such as quinoa or oats rather than pasta.

Being selective does not only applies to carbohydrates but also nutrients

How to Exercise

Physical activity, bar eating healthy, is the best thing you can do for your health. It affects your overall essence physically, *psychologically (mental health), and physiologically (internal organs). Maintaining weight or weight loss is among the many benefits of exercising. We need to incorporate walks, hikes, jogs, and other forms of working out into our daily lives. However, exercising is an activity that many of us have no time for despite our need to lose weight. This is you need to change your perception of exercise.*

First, understand that exercising is not only similar but the same as physical activity. Yes, when you spend an hour baking inside the kitchen, you have worked out. Exercising doesn't have to involve you pulling on a jogger and a running shoe. It doesn't start or end in the gym. If you find any of this difficult due to your job or lifestyle, you can still incorporate exercise into your daily routine on your weight loss journey.

Let's use these illustrations.

Since work starts at 8:30 am, wake up 2 hours early to prepare. By 8:00, you should be out of the house early. Instead of taking the bus from the bus station close to your home, walk to the next bus station; this could be 10-15minutes. Feel the morning breeze and watch the world kick start for the day. Take a bus at the next bus station to your office. Is your office space on the 3-5 floor, ignore the elevator and take the stairs instead. Done with work for the day? Take the bus or train whichever suits you and stop a few blocks or a mile from home. Walk the rest of the way home.

Going to the grocery store? Talk a walk if it is 1-2 miles away from your home. Going to see a friend or family outside your neighborhood, take the bus there, and encourage your friend or family to walk with you while you both discuss your lives. Is your friend too tired to go out?

Well, stay indoors and chat but leave a little earlier to take a brisk walk back home or halfway home.

Love cooking? Try something new during the weekends.

Now, you have worked out even without carrying that mindset with you. It is just a normal day. However, you have spent close to 30minutes exercising even without trying so hard. With this perception of working out, you don't have to beat yourself up over missing your gym sessions or not waking up early enough to jog.

In a nutshell, exercising, working out, going for that early morning run twice or thrice a week equals being physically active. Physical activity is anything that keeps you on your feet up and about. And it is easier to incorporate into your daily routine on your weight loss journey.

Leftovers Are Not Wasteful

Do you feel the need to clean your plate because you might end up feeling guilty wasting food, even if you end up overeating? Thus, making it harder to lose weight.

Growing up, our parents might have ingrained in our heads that you have to eat everything on our plates as leftovers are signs that you are either not grateful or you don't care for people starving to death.

Therefore, with or without our parents around, we eat what we don't even want. For weight loss, this food psychology is counter-productive. Whether you choose to force it down your throat or scrap it into a waste bin, this unwanted food won't help you or anyone. Forcing it down your throat will only gain you more weight or make it difficult to lose some.

For your sake, you need to

change your understanding of leftovers. What you need to do instead is to prepare a meal you can finish. Or, put less food on your plate. Change your plate size if you feel the urge to load up your plate still. If you choose to eat out, tell the waiter to wrap the leftovers to take home with you. In any case, you won't be eating it, give it to someone on the street.

With any of this, you know you are keeping to your values at the same creating a new perception of it.

We have gone through some major concepts as regards weight loss. The idea behind this chapter is to challenge what we already know about weight loss. As you can see, each relates to our perception and not necessarily an action you need to implement toward losing weight. Weight loss starts from the mind and progresses with it. Examining all we know about losing weight helps us break the restrictions put in place by fad diets, making it hard to shed those extra pounds. You can lose weight without trying so hard. All you need is to align your mindset; your body needs with your weight loss plan.

Revisiting Your Concept of Weight Loss: Making New Conclusions

While examining all you know about weight loss is important, what comes next is crucial: make new conclusions from the knowledge. You have to be open to accepting some facts and debunking some more. There are loads of information on the internet, and making new conclusions is more challenging. It goes beyond acknowledging these pieces of information to conceding it better to complement your weight loss plan.

Yes, you need to cut carbs

simultaneously, cut calories, not ignore the former in a bid for the later, but how does this help? How is this relevant?

As I said, weight loss starts from the mind; once your mind accepts an idea, your body reflects the perceptions. The whole idea of Chapter 1 is to give your mind the right information to work with and not made up ones that work selectively.

Now, let's get right into business: how can you make new conclusions towards transforming your mindset about losing weight?

Mindset Shift

Discover Your Motivation

Why are you on a weight loss program?

Discovering your motivation will help you set your mindset right towards losing weight. Know that the question doesn't have either a right or wrong answer. Each of us is permitted to have our reasons, however weird, in wanting to lose weight. Is it improved energy? Health? Increased confidence? Become more beautiful? Whichever, it still works. So, whatever your motivation is, don't fault it or allow anyone to do that to you. However, keep in mind that discovering your motivation is tied to following your weight loss plan all through. Weight loss is challenging and demands effort. Knowing if you should either lose weight or fat is a step; going further to stay motivated will keep you on the side.

Now, take a pen and write down the many reasons you want to lose weight. You can go beyond that and pin down why you identify that reason.

For instance, you feel your beauty is tied to weight loss; why?

Dig deeper into your inspiration and discover why losing weight is what you need. Once this is clear, you can be confident that whatever challenge like Thanksgiving or Christmas comes your way, you will still watch what you eat towards weight loss.

Change your goals

You might have a specific goal weight but a result and not your goal. Your goals should be realistic, small, sustainable accomplishments, which you must have complete control over. NYC-based therapist Paul Hokemeyer hinted at something like this.

Were you able to follow your menu for just 2 days? That there is a goal checked off the list. Did *you take the stairs throughout the week, shrugging off the appeal of the elevator? That's another realistic goal achieved that you have full control over.*

Most people tend to use the scale to set a weight loss goal. This makes sense because the number on the scale represents how close you are to your objective or how far out you are. However, there is a problem. What happens when you don't have the motivation to push ahead, the mindset to believe that you could reach your goal weight? These are factors that are likely to push off a weight loss plan.

Like discovering your motivation, you need to restructure your goals. These are mindset shifts that do not require any physical activity other than taking mental notes that positively transform your weight loss plan. So instead of setting a goal weight, which you have little control over, set goals like these:

Take a walk twice in 2 days.

Drink 8 liters of water

for 3 days in a row.

Eat veggies or fruits

every day for 5 days.

Stay away from your favorite fast food, cooking at home for a week.

These are realistic and actionable goals that would lead to weight loss through consistency. And the best part of it is that you have full control over it. You can beat yourself up knowing that you could have done something but choose not to or find it difficult. With the scale, the numbers are something you can only do but guess. Change your goals, a mindset shift that will reflect your weight loss plan in a good way.

Positivity

Being around positive people has

an indirect effect on your weight loss. With these kinds of individuals, you get more encouragement and excel in an emotionally healthy environment. You don't need someone who tells you, you have maybe lost a pound or two after weeks of hard work. No, they don't have to tell lies to make you feel good about yourself. Weight loss has a physical, physiological, and psychological effect on a person.

In such circumstances, you can affect someone psychologically, which prompts physical (junk eating spree, starvation) and physiological (obesity, heart problems, ulcer, anorexia). Hence, you don't need negative people around. Seek out positive people and like Chicago-based Nike NTC master trainer and run coach Emily Hutchins says, "Don't be afraid to ask for help or support."

Be in control

On "Change your goal," we have seen a little of how you being in control is important for weight loss. Have you ever craved a big bowl of your favorite ice-cream? Or let's be more realistic, a small cone of your favorite strawberry ice-cream? It got to you so bad that you just went ahead with it anyway. I mean, a cone won't suddenly propel your weight to the sky, right? No, it won't, *but you just lost one important factor that will help you lose weight: being in control. It would be best if you were in control of what you choose to eat, how and when you eat it.*

Being in control keeps you on track. Like every other mindset shift we have discussed so far, and this control is a mental prowess that indirectly impacts a weight loss program. This also includes eliminating excuses; "I am tired"; "I need a break." Being in control holds you responsible for your actions and hence, more reasons to keep to that meal plan.

Give yourself a treat

While you strive to accomplish a goal, and eventually get it, give yourself a treat now and then. No, I don't mean stuff yourself with a bowl of ice-cream. You could break a goal into milestones as they keep you on track towards your goal. With every milestone ticked off the list, celebrate yourself.

No need to do something over the top. At the same time, it should be a treat that you will enjoy and look forward to. I should be something that gets you excited enough that inspires you to stay on track and achieve that milestone. As I said, a bowl of ice-cream won't work as that deviates from your plan. Watching Netflix all day is one or taking a day off work or study is another. These are things I would gladly treat myself too. However, treats should be unique to your needs. The most important thing is that these treats do not put you off track even if it is for a moment. Towards weight loss, discipline, and control will help you reach your goals faster.

Initially, avoid the scale at all costs!

We have learned how using a weight scale to measure your progress is a bad idea. You can't control the numbers that you will see when you step on that platform. However, you can control what you eat, how you eat, and what implementations you put in place that helps you to achieve your goal.

Know that using the scale isn't exactly a terrible idea but most of us have attached its relevance to how we live our lives. In most cases, we associate them with self-destructive feelings and actions. You can use the scale if it has no effect on you but if otherwise, avoid the scale at all cost. Hokemeyer adds that you should avoid until you get to a place that the number displaying on the scale does not define your self-worth.

Mindset shift begins the process of using your mind to transform your weight loss plans. In the subsequent chapters, we will learn some unique mind-related concepts and how you can usethem to improve your plan.

Utilizing the Concept of Law of Attraction for Weight Loss

When I was about to begin my weight loss journey, I thought it was only about skipping meals, spending hours at the gym, and running five lapses around the park each morning. At the end of each day, I'd stand on my scale, expecting to have lost some pounds. It worried me when I'd see the same result for days. I was this close to giving up because I felt, "What's the use of starving myself when I'm getting no results?"

I just wanted to shed some fat, and I wanted to move my body *freely, I wanted to stand up tall in gatherings, I wanted my jeans to fit, and wanted to slim down.*

Yes, I wanted all these, but I didn't put my mind to losing weight. All the things I did, the running and going to the gym, were just hurdles I felt I needed to cross, and ta-dah, I'd be slim! But you know what, I was wrong. To achieve anything at all in life, you have to set your mind to it, this is what I soon learned. You have to stop saying to yourself, "I'm fat" or "I'm overweight" and start believing that you can lose weight if you set your mind to it.

In all my years in college, no one ever really taught me this. All I heard was, "Think it, believe it, achieve it" and I didn't even know there was more to this and there was something called the Law of Attraction. This was an eye-opener for me, and my weight loss journey began when I found this out.

The Law of Attraction

This law is the ability to attract into your life whatever it is you put your mind to. The law states that you get whatever it is you're determined to achieve, that your thoughts will transform into reality.

You may be thinking this is some religious ideology that doesn't make any actual sense but, it has been scientifically proven.

The section of the brain involved with 'intention' is connected to that involved with 'action' so, when you kick-start your intention section, you're kick-starting your action region. However, for action to take place, your intention has to be strong. The Law of Attraction doesn't mean that if you think of having a Ferrari, a Ferrari is just going to appear in front of you. If that's what you're thinking, you're getting it all wrong.

What it is stating is that we make things happen when we intend to do them when we set our minds to do them.

Sadly, only some people are aware that we attract what we have put out there at every moment of our existence. It's like some magnet of some sort, attracting only what we send out. This means that if your mind is trained on negative thoughts alone, you will get negative returns, and if you have positive goals, you are willing to achieve, you are going to achieve them.

There's something Bob Proctor, a teacher of Law of Attraction, said one time, "No one can cause you to think something you don't want to think. That's where we can choose..."

Proctor is saying that you have so many choices; you have the choice of what to think, what to hear, or how to look. So, I'm asking you right now, how do you want to look? This is a question I constantly asked myself as I began to embrace the Law of Attraction's concept. I was hoping you could ask yourself this question and give an answer before moving on to the next part.

How Does the Law of Attraction Help with Weight Loss?

Now, the purpose of all my long talk about this law is to understand that everything you want to achieve starts in your mind. I want you to understand that the journey of losing weight doesn't start at the gym door or with eating only a slice of apple for breakfast. It starts in your mind. It begins with you

visualizing your success and believing that you can do it.
Here are the steps I took when I decided to utilize the Law of Attraction for my weight loss journey.

Ask Yourself Why You Want to Lose Weight

For me, I was tired of my body, feeling like a sack of sand and having to drag myself around. That was why I decided to lose some weight. What is it for you? Why do you want to go on this journey?

Even if we want to go by the simple "think it, believe it, and achieve it" concept, you have to go through the first stage, which *is the "think" stage. So think about why you want to do this.*

But I must warn you. Your reasons for wanting to lose weight shouldn't come from a place of self-loathing or from comparing yourself to others. Your reason should be from a desire to grow and from self-respect. If you are comfortable with your size, don't try to change it for anyone! Trust me, it's not worth it.

Build the Image of What You Want to Look Like

As you are at this point, I'm hoping you've answered the question of how you want to look. Before you even begin with a weight loss plan, picture how you want your body to be and ask yourself why you want to be that way.

Bob Proctor inspired me throughout my weight loss journey. I read his books and watched his lessons on YouTube, and from one of them, I learned that you have to stop focusing on present unwanted circumstances and focus instead on what you want.

You have to stop repeating, "I'm fat" and start saying to yourself things like, "I know I can be slim" or "I have to work towards being slim." Keep this simple sequence in mind: thoughts turn to feelings, feelings turn to actions, and actions turn to results.

This means that in the long run,

your thoughts revolve into becoming your results. Here's what Oprah Winfrey said, "Create the highest, grandest vision possible for your life because you become what you believe."

Internalize This Image, Increase Your Self-Awareness

When you think of how you want to look at the end of your weight loss journey, you must internalize this image. Proctor explains that to attract what you want, your thoughts must be accompanied by a deep desire. Become enthusiastic about it, dwell on it; keep thinking about this image.

Moreover, thinking about this image is not enough. You have to start thinking of yourself as fit, active, and vibrant. Think of yourself as someone who has already lost a hundred pounds while in the gym. When jogging past a lady in skinny jeans, think of yourself as someone who those jeans will fit. You wouldn't know when it actually would!

Even Lady Gaga has experimented with this, and she says, "Constantly remind yourself of the person you are destined to become... Before you realize it, the mindset and the actions you implemented will produce the results you desire".

Meditation

I went through all the processes I've listed, but this one did it for me. Through the help of this free meditation, Millionaire Meditation, I was able to reprogram my mind and way of thinking.

This is the program that taught me everything I needed to know at that time.

I graduated from college, and walking down that floor to get my degree was a memorable moment. The six years I spent in college taught me nothing as important as the information I am sharing with you today. I'll go into this meditation technique in the next chapter.

Get That Body!

You can only attract the energy that is in harmony with the thoughts you have internalized. What I'm simply saying is, with all the measures above, you should have successfully internalized the image you want to be and backed it up with actions and words of affirmation. And so long as your mind and your body agree on a certain goal or desire, you are going to achieve it.

Proctor said once that, "We can create the life that we want, we can put ourselves into the vibration that we have to be in to attract what we want to attract."

About losing weight, this means that you can choose how you want to look, you can internalize that image, and definitely, you can attract that image.

Even Idris Elba believes this simple trick. Here's what he said about it, "I think my imagination has always kept me going. I just imagined myself collecting awards. I just imagined myself getting big parts. That's part of my inner magic. If I can see myself doing it, I can do it."

These are some of the techniques that I still use to this day to create the life that I want. They are not only how I attract wealth, but how I keep my body in shape.

Now that you know what's preventing you from completing your weight loss journey, it's time for you to change your mindset. There are effective ways to do this, which I've already listed, like meditations, words of affirmation, and visualization. The successive chapters will go into more detail about them.

I tried out all these processes because I wanted my success to be guaranteed. I believed so much in the Law of Attraction, and sure enough, I got the body that I wanted.

Give this your best shot. Set your

mind to it. Believe you can get the body that you want. Repeat words of affirmation to yourself. Like 50 Cent did, convince yourself you're going to make it regardless of what people think! You can do it!

Practical Ways of Connecting Your Mind and Body: Meditation

In the previous chapter, I listed the processes through which the Law of Attraction helped me in my weight loss journey. One of the ways I mentioned was meditation, and as I said before, this was how I got the majority of the assistance for my weight loss journey.

Why do you need to connect your mind and body? I know this is a question you may be asking; but, don't you worry, I have an answer for you. You need to connect your mind and body because your feelings, thoughts, and emotions can affect your health and also your physical appearance. They can affect your body posture, your body size, and *how you carry yourself. In simpler terms, the mind impacts the body, and the body affects the mind. This is why there is a big need for you to connect your mind and your body.*

I want you to understand that losing weight doesn't happen in the blink of an eye. It takes time, work, determination, and courage. Although the Law of Attraction states that you can get anything you want, you have to set your mind on it diligently.

It's the same with weight loss. If you want to lose some pounds, you have to believe that you are capable of doing it, you have to discipline yourself, keep in mind that body you want to have, and

work towards getting that body.
And one way to perfectly create
that image that you want for
yourself and accept and love your
body is through meditation.
Many people underestimate the
power of meditation, and to them,
it's just sitting with your legs
folded under you, your eyes
closed, and repeating, "hmm."
I'm telling you today that that
isn't all there is to meditation. For
me, it helps to be in tune with my
spirit. Those few minutes of quiet
grant you this inner peace and
self-appreciation you will get
from nowhere else.

What is Meditation All About

Before I go further, I'd like to
answer the question of what

meditation is. You probably already know what it is, but I'd like to give it my definition. Meditation is a practice for wellness proven repeatedly to reduce stress, redeem focus, improve self-esteem, and is beneficial to physical and mental health.

It is by no mistake that of the four ways of connecting your mind and body, meditation is the first that I discuss. I'm not implying that it is the only effective or the essential process; rather, it is the process that helped me when I was on my weight loss journey.

Why Should You Meditate?

Before telling you my meditation process and how the Millionaire Meditation program helped, you should know the benefits of meditation and the important role it can play on your weight loss journey. You should meditate because:

- *It relaxes your nerves.*
- *It increases your self-awareness and self-acceptance.*
- *It reduces stress and anxiety.*
- *It keeps you healthy because it boosts your immune system.*
- *It improves sleep. Yes, meditation shortens the time it takes to fall asleep and also increases the quality of sleep.*

- *Most importantly, for you, it improves metabolism and assists in weight loss.*

Getting Started

Now I'm hoping you understand the usefulness of meditation in your weight loss journey. What you are probably wondering now is how you, too, can take control of your mind. Like I've said before, there are many ways for you to do this (which I'll be taking my time to explain in full details to you). However, I want to tell you how the Millionaire Meditation program taught me everything and changed my life for the better.

The man, Wesley Virgin, quickly became my mentor, and I listened to everything he would tell me because he's a multi-millionaire, and I trusted that he knew what he was talking about. While this program focuses on making money, it also applies to every aspect of life. Whatever it is you are looking for to achieve, you get all the techniques I used and still use to achieve my biggest goals from the program.

He has created a mindset hacking system that will show you how to change your way of thinking, and when you do this, you will be able to look at things in a more positive light. Do you know what the good news is? These mind hacks are available in a PDF and audio file, and if you are a visual learner (like me), you are not left out as the program also comes in a video format. The program's main message is that you need the right mindset to succeed in anything in life. This is why I'm so intent on you checking it out. If it worked for me, it definitely would for you.

Let's briefly talk about overeating. An average of plus-sized people over-eats to avoid stress, and if this is something you can relate to, you are not alone. Emotional eating is when people eat too much due to some strong emotions that outweigh their physical feelings of fullness. To *help with this, there is a need for mindful eating and meditation.*

By mindful eating, I mean eating because you are hungry and not because you are feeling overwhelmed or stressed out. Mindful eating helps reduce emotional eating but, while it can lead to weight loss, losing weight should not be your primary motivation for doing it. Because once your food choices are based on some physical outcome, you are expecting, it is no longer mindful eating.

Meditation, on the other hand, also plays a vital role in the weight loss process because it helps to reduce stress. Remember, stress leads to overeating, and overeating leads to gaining a whole lot of weight. If the stress, which is the trigger, can be eradicated, you are on the first step of your weight loss journey. So, these are the ways meditation will help you control your mind and how you eat:

It will help remove

that guilt for those

who struggle with

overeating. It will

help you recognize

if you're eating

due to stress or

hunger.

It is guaranteed to make your weight loss efforts long-lasting. Meditation gives you that drive to stick to your diet and exercise routine.

It helps you control your

emotions and also your cravings.

So, it is right to say it disciplines

you! And as always, it reduces the

stress and anxiety that comes

with trying to lose weight.

Now let's head on to the meditation process. Many people get anxious at the thought of meditating because they feel they cannot do it. Are you one of these people? Meditation is not extraordinary as you may think it to be; it's just a simple practice for the mind's wellness. Even just a few minutes of relaxing and breathing is a form of meditation as it can relax your mind and increase your focus.

While meditation has various forms and benefits, I'll focus on mindfulness meditation, which encourages you to eradicate negative thoughts and put positive ones in their place.

The first step is to set aside a place for meditating because you will build a special feeling there, and it will make you get into the meditative spirit easily.

Sit comfortably with your feet on

the floor and your back supported. Make sure you are in a comfortable and relaxing position.

Close your eyes, and keep them close. You don't want anything distracting you.

Focus on nothing else but your breathing. Focus on the rising and falling of your chest and go at a slow and steady pace, inhaling and breathing out comfortable breaths.

Now is the time for you to invite into your mind healing and beautiful breaths into your body. By this, I mean that you invite in love and peace into your heart. Love for the body you have now and peace with it. You envisage that dream body you want to have. Remember, no pressure, no tension. It's all love.

Keep up with this for as long as you like; you may set a timer if you wish. When you gently open your eyes, there's going to be nothing but positive energy flowing through you.

Meditation is not your ultimate guarantee of weight loss. Don't go thinking that you'll start losing weight if you meditate daily. No, that's not the message I'm trying to pass across. It doesn't replace your dieting or exercising plan; rather, it supports these positive changes so long as you do it with determination and patience.

Meditation allows you to challenge your limiting beliefs and helps you think of what you want for your body and mind. While meditating, you can explore your motivations for weight loss and seek the truth of why you skip your routines all the time or why it's so difficult to get yourself out of bed to go for a run. I'm telling you all these because they are things I've been through. Till today, I still meditate even though I have the body that I've always wanted. To get that body you want, give it a shot, connect your mind and body first, and see how everything else turns out.

Practical Ways of Connecting Your Mind and Body: Visualization

Psychologists have long proven that the images you create in your mind can have a strong effect on your body. In the previous chapter, I introduced you to the first process to connect your body and mind, which is meditation. Although meditation was the technique that helped me through my weight loss journey, the potency of visualization cannot be overemphasized.

Before going further into this book, I want you to understand that there is no 'best' way to lose weight. Rather, there are so many ways to go about it, and anyone of them can work for you.

However, one thing you should note (I know I've said this about a million times already) is that you have to connect your thoughts (or mind) and your body. You need to go deep into your thoughts and create this image of yourself that you want. I mentioned this as the fifth step of the meditation process in the last chapter, and it is called visualize.

What is Visualization All About

For me, visualization is the process of focusing your thoughts on circumstances, behaviors, or events you want to happen. It is the act of forming a picture of somebody/something in your mind.

This idea is based on the belief that your mind and body are connected. That by creating a detailed image of what you want and visualizing it time and time again, there is a high chance you are going to get it. Through filling your mind with positive thoughts, visualization can have a physical effect on your body. This mental trick helps you imagine how great that goal you want to meet (which in your case is to be in good shape) will be and will make any hard work (dieting or working out) you may have to go through to get it (the body) worth it.

Just like some people think meditation is some weird

religious ideology, some think the idea of visualization is a little off the roof. Well, if you need some reassurance, let me let you know that it has been tested and proven by scientists. Stephen Kosslyn, the author of Top Brain, Bottom Brain, explains that "Visualization activates the same neural networks that actual task performance does, which can strengthen the connection between brain and body."

The mind doesn't know the difference between what is imagined and what is reality. So, when you visualize yourself as fit and slim, your mind encodes this as if you are!

How Visualization Can Help with Weight Loss

Do you know that many people have used visualization to heal and move past challenges or conditions such as asthma, insomnia, and even anxiety? Or that athletes, let's say soccer players, use visualization to picture the goals they are going to score? Visualization is this tool, just like the Law of Attraction, that many people use without knowing they are using it. When you see yourself getting an A in English at the beginning of the school year, that's visualization. When you picture your legs fitting into those skinny jeans or your flat tummy looking great in that dress, that's visualization.

For weight loss, there are so many areas visualization can help you with. It helps with motivation, to boost workouts, to build confidence, to increase self-love, for healthy eating, and to overcome bad habits. Here are two benefits, among many others, I got from visualization throughout my weight loss journey, which I'm sure you're going to get if you try it out:

- *It helped to overcome my inner battles*

Losing weight is hard when you have self-destructive thoughts flowing through your head. It is hard when you feel lazy all the time, avoid your exercise routines or overeat. I struggled with all these, finding it hard to get myself up and begin my routines or follow my dieting plan. But, when I started to visualize the body I wanted, I disciplined myself to do all I needed to do. Because I realized every work I had to do was going to be worth it soon enough.

- *It kept me going*

Because I had that body, I wanted to be stuck in my mind, and I couldn't stop going. Eating the same foods day after day and spending hours in the gym sometimes got me tired, but whenever that body came up in my mind, I'd get myself up and get myself going. Visualization is just like medicine for low motivation.

Getting Started

Now, we have covered what visualization is and the benefits you are sure to gain from it. The next thing you need to know is how to get started. Visualization is not so much of a big deal and is not something you need to be taught to do, but, because this book is an ultimate guide to weight loss and I've promised to be of help to you throughout your weight loss journey, I'll be sharing some techniques I used *for myself.*

Visualize that body as you want it to be I've been repeating this since the first page of this book, and trust me; you're going to see more of it as you go on. I'm not going to give you tips like close your eyes and breathe slowly. If you're visualizing during meditation then, that's fine. But, four or five times a day, maybe when you wake up or as you walk down the street, think about that slim body you wish to have. See yourself in a bikini or shirtless at the beach. Picture yourself in those places you've always wanted to go to, your high school reunion, maybe. Create your new reality; imagine how beautiful or handsome you will look.

Imagine yourself eating healthier foods. The first thing to do for this is to consider what your eating goals are. Do you want to stop emotional eating (we discussed this in the previous chapter)? Do you want to eat less sugar? Do you want to reduce your food portions? Whichever of this is the eating goal you want to achieve, start visualizing yourself accomplishing this goal.

Imagine yourself satisfied with smaller portions of food. See yourself enjoying a plate of salad or veggies instead of a bar of chocolate. Visualize yourself shopping for carrots instead of candies, and before

you know it, you're good to go.
Visualize your workout sessions
I'm hoping you are not a lazy ass
as I was. Well, if you are,
visualization can be of help to
you as it was to me. It has been
proven scientifically that your
physical performance can
increase by visualizing yourself
performing this activity. Like I
said before, this is the trick
athletes use. This can be done by
visualizing yourself feeling good
about your workouts or going
through your routine in your
mind. Feel your muscles
working as they would during
the actual workout, and before
you know it, you will be fast
becoming fitter than you would

normally.

Visualize receiving compliments

*One definite thing is that people
who care about you, friends,
and family will acknowledge
your efforts to lose weight and
encourage you as you go on.
However, there's no harm in
visualizing them completing you
about how sexy or gorgeous
your body looks, or is there?
Imagine walking down the street
and your neighbor saying, "I
love how your legs look in those
jeans." Imagine your colleague
asking for your workout routine
because he wants to look like
you. Imagine your mum getting
you this skimpy dress and
saying, "I knew instantly this*

dress was going to fit!" Go ahead
and build various scenarios in
your mind; no one's stopping
you.

Runaway from negativity

When I started visualizing how I
wanted my body to look, there
were these thoughts that resided
at the back of my mind. Thoughts
like I was kidding myself or like,
"there's no way this would work,
you're just being a fool." These
thoughts were doing nothing but
destroying all the work I'd done.
So, what I started to do was
ignore those thoughts. Whenever
they tried to creep into my mind,
I cast them out. Do not let
disbelief crawl into your mind.
We've talked about how you

should remove words like "I'm fat" from your vocabulary. There's simply no space for negativity on your weight loss journey.

You might face challenges like procrastination or distraction with visualization but how to overcome them is to remind yourself of the result you are hoping to get and knowing that you will be happy when you get this result. For distractions, visualize when you know you are less likely to be disturbed, maybe immediately you wake up or at night before you sleep.

One last thing I want you to know is that visualization is not fantasizing; neither is it being over-optimistic. Visualization is not hanging pictures of Jennifer Lopez on your wall and wishing to be like her. It is having personal goals for yourself and not comparing yourself to anybody. It is also not sitting in a place all day and dreaming of having a great body. It aims high but acknowledging that there are hurdles and challenges you must overcome to get that body.

You need to be consistent with visualization. The more you do it, the better you feel, and the faster you begin to see results. Cheer yourself on each day and be your number one fan. I'm sure you can do it because it's something I went through myself. And surely, if I could do it, you most definitely can!

Practical Ways of Connecting Your Mind and Body: Affirmations

To get anything in this world, you have to be one hundred percent determined to get it. It may take you days or months or years to achieve, but only to stay determined till the end will give you the results you need. In your case, what you want to achieve is losing weight, and once you embrace and believe this change is possible, this change is going to happen.

Research shows that about 45,000 to 51,000 thoughts cross our minds each day. This means that in a minute, you could think about

250 different things! What is, however, sad is that about 75% of these thoughts are negative. In a minute, you could be thinking about how you'll look odd at the reunion, how you friends are ashamed of you, how you wouldn't get that job because of your size, how you're wasting your time at the gym, or how your partner is ashamed to take you out. That's a whole lot of negativity!

One way to overcome these doubts and fears that you can never get that slim or fit body is through positive affirmations.

What Do Affirmations Mean in Weight Loss?

Affirmations are short statements that are positive and geared towards a specific thought or belief. These statements are to be repeated to oneself or written down from time to time. The sentences are to be positive, specific, and in the present tense.

Simply put, affirmations refer to a practice of self-empowerment or positive thinking with the belief that anything can be achieved through this.

They are aimed to affect the subconscious and the conscious mind and awaken inspiring and motivating mental images. According to those statements you affirmed, these affirmations and the images that have been brought up are etched on the subconscious mind and result in changes in habits, behavior, or actions.

For weight loss, affirmations mean the same thing. It is taking charge of your thoughts and channeling them into positivity. It is removing from your mind statements like, "I am fat." It is reassuring yourself that you can stick to your diet plan. It is having a confident mindset that you will succeed in your quest for weight loss.

Repeating affirmations to yourself doesn't mean you should pretend like you've got everything under control when you don't do. Rather, it is to make you feel sure, certain, and strengthen your confidence level to achieve your weight loss goals.

Some Weight Loss Affirmations to Help You

These are some of the positive affirmations I used during my weight loss journey to reprogram my mind and to keep me focused on the goals I wanted to achieve.
"I love my body."
"I am getting fitter and stronger every day." "I look and feel great."
"I love to exercise regularly."
"I love how healthy food tastes."
"I am already achieving my weight loss goals."
"I only eat when I'm hungry and not when I'm stressed out." "I'm on my way to developing an attractive body."

"I am a weight loss story success."
"I am a beautiful/handsome person."
"I find losing weight very easy and natural." "I eat a lot of veggies and fruit."
"I deserve to be healthy, to be slim and to be beautiful/handsome."

How Affirmations Can Help in Weight Loss

You should know that you are what you think you are, and your life is a reflection of your thoughts. If all you think about yourself is that you are fat looking in the mirror, you're going to see a fat lady or a fat man. But, if you think that you are strong and capable of achieving what you want or fulfilling your weight loss goals when you look in the mirror, you'll see a strong woman or a strong man. This is the power of affirmations and let's looks deeper into what affirmations can do for you.

Affirmations motivate you
I've already said this about a hundred times. When you constantly repeat words like, "I am a weight loss success story," do you think you're going to give up? Of course not! No way can happen because you cannot be a success story if you don't complete those goals. So, the more you repeat these statements, the more motivated you are to make them become your reality. I did this and look at

where I am today; I am a weight loss success story!

Affirmations influence the subconscious and take over.

What do I mean by taking over? I mean, they will overpower negative thoughts. They will rule your subconscious and lead you in the path to follow. Thoughts like "I am overweight" will be overshadowed with thoughts like "I look and feel great." Your positive thoughts will overtake, and just like magic, your body will get to work!

Affirmations keep you focused on your weight loss goals.

When you've got words like, "I love to exercise regularly" pinned

on your wall; you're going to
want to exercise. That's the power
of affirmations; you can't ignore
it! When you fill your head with
only positive thoughts supporting
the goal you want to achieve,
they will always be present,
reminding you of the things
you've got to do.

Affirmations change your mindset and behavior:

This is very similar to the point,
as mentioned earlier. When you
begin to think positively about
yourself, consciously or
unconsciously, you are going to
change. When you say to
yourself, "I love my body," your
self-esteem is going to increase,
and when you walk, you're
going to do so with your head

high. *If your head is filled with positive thoughts, you're going to smile more, and you're going to be happy. People around you will notice this change, and you may even attract more people into your life.*

Getting Started
In the last chapter, we talked about visualization, and when I talked about getting started, I mentioned visualizing yourself being slim and working out and getting compliments. An affirmation, on the other hand, isn't about visualizing but about professing. That is, it is about saying or writing what you want for yourself. Here some tips you need to get started.

Let go of negative beliefs.
You may have beliefs about
yourself living rent-free in your
head and going with you
wherever you go. Some of these
beliefs may be things people
have said to you at one time or
the other like, "You can't
possibly lose all that fat" or "You
can't achieve anything."
Someone said this to me once,
and it was hard, but I had to let it
go. There was no way my
affirmations could be effective if
I didn't let go of that belief. I want
you to do the same and to clear
your mind of every form of
negativity.

Focus on one goal at a time
I want to believe your goal is to
lose weight, and that is why
you're reading this book now.
So, your affirmations should be
centered around what you want
for your body. I have helped you
with some affirmative
statements already, and you can
also make some for yourself.
Your statements should be in the
present tense and not in future
tense because those things are
what you want for yourself
nowbecause that's who you want
to be seen in the mirror now.
Reciting your affirmations in
front of a mirror is advisable
because you'll be looking at
yourself and reassuring yourself

and motivating yourself.

Use affirmations that feel natural to you You don't have to use the ones I gave you or the ones you find on the Internet. It's your weight loss journey, not anyone else's. For example, if you don't feel comfortable with saying, "I love how healthy food tastes" because it's not true and you don't love the taste, say something like, "I am open to enjoying healthy food." That's positive thinking, isn't it? Focus on the things you want and not on the things you don't want. Instead of saying, "I don't want to sleep past my jogging time," say, "I am capable of waking up early to go for my run." I also advise that you start your statements with "I am" as much as possible because whatever we think we are, we become.

Be consistent
This is not a "one-day" thing. You should repeat your words of affirmation as much as you can, every day. It is advisable to do so at least twice a day: in the morning, you wake up and at night before you go to sleep. Challenge yourself and make a 30-day commitment plan to repeat your affirmations for each of the days. Promise me you'll stick to this plan no matter what. I believe in you and hoping you will do it.
These affirmations should always be present in your

thoughts. Repeat them in front of your mirror in the morning, repeat them in the shower, repeat them while you are driving, repeat them in bed, and always have them in mind! Write them down on post-it notes and leave them in different places, in your room, your desk at work, your refrigerator, or in your notebooks. And remember, if you think these affirmations will work, they will, and if you think they won't work, they won't because whatever it is, you're thinking it is working.

Practical Ways of Connecting Your Mind and Body: Scripting

Scripting is the last method of connecting your mind and body that I'm going to be discussing in this book, and truth be told, all the methods are interconnected. All of them have many similarities, the major ones being that they are all Law of Attraction techniques, and all of them require positive thoughts. Visualization talks about conjuring in your head, positive images, and thoughts about that body you want. Affirmations are about professing positive words and statements about the life you want to live and who you want to be. And now, scripting is *about writing down these positive thoughts and images you have for yourself.*

What is Scripting All About Scripting is a technique that involves writing down the reality that you want. Instead of saying it to yourself as affirmations require you to do, scripting is all about writing it down. It involves your imaginations taking control (positively, of course) and communicating them through words written down in a story-like kind of way.

In the previous chapter, I mentioned how you should write affirmations on post-it notes and place them on the desks and refrigerators, right? Well, that is scripting. We can say that affirmation is the oral form of visualization, and scripting is the written form!

Scripting reminds me of those days as children when we'd fantasize about our future partners or how we'd be Cinderella or find a girl like Cinderella, and we'd write down these fantasies. Why scripting is different from this is because, in its case, you're writing about your reality that is yet to happen.

How Scripting Can Help in Weight Loss

Like visualization and affirmations, scripting helped me in my journey. I'd stay in my room writing and writing about myself being slim and the things I'd do when I get slim and about the way people would admire me and about how I'd walk past that lady that once told me I'd never lost weight. I wrote about all the things and now, look where I am! I'm a weight-loss testimony, and I'm writing my book! These are some of the benefits of scripting for weight loss that you should know:

It allows you to translate your visualization into word form: I've already said this, that *scripting is the written form of visualization. Some people express themselves better when they write, and if you're such a person, scripting will be great for you. You have the freedom to write as much as you want about the future you want; about the body you want. For those who struggle to visualize or speak words of affirmations to themselves mentally, this is a great alternative.*

It allows you to explore your goals in details.

Do you read books, like novels? If you do, you'd know how detailed the writers' descriptions always are. Do you know how they go on to describe everything in a room from the ceiling to the foot mat? It's the same thing with scripting. You are free to explore and to go into specific details about your dreams and desires and exactly how you want to be. This is going to motivate you to keep up with your routines anytime you read them.

It allows you to believe in the process. Have you ever gone through pages of your past diaries and found where you wrote that you needed something desperately, something that you got later on? That's how it is going to be with scripting. Imagine coming across the scripts you write now in five years when you're all slim and sexy. You're going to be like, "Oh! This thing worked!" and you're going to want to tell people about the process the same way I'm telling you to know. It's going to feel like you predicted the future!

Getting Started

Like all the other processes of connecting your body and your mind, scripting is personal, and *no one should teach you how to go about it. Being a technique doesn't make it a "task," and so you can go about it anyway of your choice. However, there are few things you should know, especially if you are just hearing about scripting for the first time. Before you begin scripting, take a moment to think about the relationship you have with your body. How do you feel about it? How well do you take care of it? What measures have you put in place for losing weight? How well are you ready to embrace dieting and exercising? After you have considered all these, go ahead and begin. These are some things you should know:*

It should be in the present tense.

Like affirmations, scripting should be written in the present tense because it gives the feeling that that body is already yours. This may be a bit difficult to write, and you might end up with so many grammatical mistakes because you are writing about a future event in the present tense. Well, it's not an English essay, and no one's going to grade you. You're to write in the present tense because that allows you to connect deeply with those goals. So, whether you make blunders or not, be sure to be connected to what you're writing while you're writing it.

Express gratitude for the body you have right now
You don't need to write this down; all you need to do is to take a few moments to breathe and ask yourself the things you love about the body you have known and why you're grateful for it. This is necessary because if you are sincerely grateful for the body, you have now, you will attract a body you'll be even more grateful for. On the other hand, you can also write, expressing gratitude for the body you want and are sure you are going to get.

It should be clear and precise.

One way to make this easier for you is to put yourself in the shoes of your future self and write like you're writing at that future time you like to achieve your goal. For example, if you wish to have gotten your dream body by Christmas, you can start scripting like this, "It is Christmas and the whole family is home. I am in my pink skimpy dress...." Or do you wish to have gotten the body before the class reunion? You can start in the same way. The more details you can write down, the more powerful your manifestation is going to be. Go all in and bring your vision to life. It is yourvision; make it as grand as possible!

It should involve emotions.

As you have put yourself in the shoes of your future self, you are also supposed to feel the emotions of them. This means that you are supposed to feel amazing and happy. Feel like you would during the class reunion or at the family Christmas dinner. The statements you write down are supposed to make you feel excited, powerful, and alive.

If they don't, don't bother putting them on your refrigerator or desk.

Focus on what you want and not what you don't

Please, do not write down things like, "I am no longer fat" or "I am no longer wearing XXL clothes." This is because if you think this way, you are focused on the aspect of not wanting something rather than wanting something. Remember, this is a technique of the Law of Attraction; you are going to attract what you want and not what you don't want. So, you are supposed to channel your mind in the way of the slim body you want and not the overweight one you don't want.

It should be believable.

In Chapter 6, I told you how you shouldn't use affirmations you don't believe in. It's the same with scripting. Don't write down what you don't believe you can achieve because if you do so, the whole process is just going to be a waste of time. You can't say your body and mind are connected when you have doubts. So, try not to dream too big or write down impossible things.

Rather, write down achievable and believable goals and dreams that you are ready to work towards and accomplish.

So, we have successfully talked about the four ways of connecting your mind and your body. And you know the good news? All these methods can work for you, whether you decide to use one of them or all of them. But I strongly advise that you use all because they are certain to get you in that right and positive state of mind needed to guide you throughout your weight loss journey.

Just think of this way. You wake up in the morning and bed; you visualize the body you want and the compliments you'd receive. Then, you go into the bathroom to get yourself ready for the day, and in there, you take some time in front of the mirror to repeat some affirmations to yourself. And later on, you find yourself with a pen and paper, describing that body you want and how good about yourself it'd make you feel. Tell me, if you do all these each day, do you think negative thoughts will have a chance to reside in your mind? Not! Because by doing all these, your mind (which is occupied with positivity always) and your body would be connected and working hand in hand for that body you want.

Emotional Fitness Techniques
When you purchased this book, you might have been expecting to find only chapters talking about exercise routines and dieting plans; but, in about six chapters, I've been talking about the mind

more than I have about the body. This is because the mind controls the body; it's like the body's controlling unit. And that's why I explained to you in detail four ways of connecting the mind and body- meditation, visualization, affirmations, and scripting. Many think that physical fitness is the only requirement for weight loss; however, it is just a vital part of it just as emotional fitness is. You have to keep your mind fit the same way it is necessary to keep your body fit. Remember, we are trying to connect the two of them so one can't stay fit while the other isn't. This is why there is a need for emotional fitness, and this is what this chapter will be centered on.

What is Emotional Fitness?

In simple terms, emotional fitness is the idea that our minds need to be exercised and fit just as our bodies are. It is a state of mind where you can control your thoughts by dwelling on positive and constructive thoughts and managing to avoid negative ones. To practice those methods of connecting your mind and body, you need to be emotionally fit because, as I've said before, each of them requires positive thoughts.

It has been scientifically proven that our EQ (emotional intelligence) is more important *than our IQ, so this means that being emotionally fit is very important for our overall well-being and success.*

You are about to start a journey (weight loss journey), and you are feeling anxious and stressed about the whole thing. What if it doesn't work? What if it's just a waste of time?
How can I possibly lose all these weights? You're trying to be emotionally balanced and train your thoughts on the right and positive things.

Well, emotional fitness is the best weapon to fight these thoughts and challenge-like problems. When you're fit emotionally, nothing will seem difficult to you because you have grown the inner strength to prevent any negativity from penetrating your mind and obstructing your goal.

Elements of Emotional Fitness

There are three principles on which emotional fitness is built on. These include mindfulness, connection, and gratitude. I'll give you details about each of them to fully understand what emotional fitness entails and its usefulness in achieving your weight loss goal.

Mindfulness

To be mindful is simply to be aware. Mindfulness is your nonjudgmental and full awareness of what is happening now(of the present moment). You are a non-biased observer of your thoughts, feelings, and emotions instead of allowing them to overwhelm you. It is being fully present and engaged in whatever you are doing at the moment, without distraction or judgment.

This can be cultivated with the help of techniques like focusing on breathing or meditation. Meditation, however, is a completely different act from mindfulness because it requires you to set aside time for it, stay in a quiet place, and a comfortable position. Meditation allows us to build the skill of mindfulness so *that we can learn to apply it to our everyday life.*

Unlike meditation, mindfulness is not a temporary state that's only present for a while and then disappears for the rest of the day. Mindfulness is more like a state of living, which allows us to be fully present in any circumstance we find ourselves.

The importance of mindfulness is that by becoming aware of negative or unpleasant thoughts and emotions, you have a choice to handle them or react calmly when faced with them. You become more thoughtful in the way you deal with your emotions or anger, and the more you *practice mindfulness, the more it becomes present in your life every day.*

Connection
Some people prefer to spend time with themselves. In contrast, others are social beings and loves being around people, but your relationships affect your well-being and happiness no matter the category you fall under. When talking about emotional fitness, the connection we talk about is the feeling of belonging, the feeling of being among, or a part of something.

It's no news that having relationships in a place, like a friend at work, increases your output and level of satisfaction, and so does feeling connected to a pet or place.

Whether relationships are intimate or social, it contributes greatly to our happiness because we are social beings. Having someone who goes with you to the gym or goes for a jog with you will increase your zeal and determination to lose weight. Studies have also shown that healthy relationships and connections reduce stress, anxiety, and depression.

So, it is important to grow and nature healthy relationships with *people around you to boost your mental and emotional health.*

Gratitude

In the last chapter, I talked about how you should express gratitude for the body you have now and the one you have visualized to have in the future. Gratitude is an essential and very powerful aspect of your emotional fitness. It involves being consciously thankful and appreciative of what you have right now. It is the conscious appreciation of the body you have now, of the people who love you, of your job, of the places you love to go, of your home, and of certain opportunities or experiences you've had.

Gratitude works hand in hand

with optimism, that is, having a positive mindset about the now and the future. Gratitude exercises are quick and easy to help to improve happiness, reduce stress, and control depression. Studies have shown that one's level of thankfulness can be increased, and some of the ways to do this are by:

- *Keeping a journal where you write down what you're thankful for daily. It could be anything, from the pie you had at breakfast to the phone call from a longtime friend.*
- *Making an effort to give one compliment per day to one person*

- Having a bulletin board with pictures and words that make you feel grateful.

This should be kept in a place you can see it regularly.

- Consciously using your five senses when walking to find out what you're grateful for.

How to Improve Emotional Fitness

Now that we've talked about the three aspects of emotional fitness and their benefits, it is important to know how to incorporate them into your everyday life to improve your emotional fitness.

Be aware of how you're feeling. We've talked about mindfulness already. The question now is, *how can you become mindful at all times? How can this be done? The very step is to try to practice mindfulness, and this is paying attention to your feelings. When you do this, you send signals to your brains to manage them.*

Anytime you feel unpleasant or have such thoughts, ask yourself, "What am I reacting to?" It's okay to feel angry, afraid, or sad, but you need to take responsibility for your emotions. Analyze your thoughts and ask yourself your reason for feeling that way. That's how to take responsibility and how to be in the present moment.

Also, you have to listen to your body. Remember that your mind and body are connected, so you notice how your body reacts when you feel a certain kind of way. Becoming more aware of our emotions and having control of our attention is the essential technique for better emotional fitness.

Eliminate negative thinking with a strategy

Your thoughts determine the quality of how you feel every single time. This means that you can change how you feel about things by changing the way you think about things. Changing the way you think about your body can change the way you feel about it.

When you stop thinking you're overweight, you're

going to stop feeling you're overweight.

The first thing to do on achieving this is to identify negative talk both from you or from others. Learn what is wrong to say to oneself, for example, "I'm fat" is negative talk.

After doing this, you have to notice how you talk to yourself. That inner voice in your head, is it harsh? Is it judgmental? Or is it sarcastic? And if you find out it's anyone of this, why don't you try changing it? Learn to talk to yourself calmly or emphatically. Even when you're criticizing yourself, do it as gently as you can. Even if no one is your friend, *you have to be your friend, don't you?*

Build a strong relationship with your emotions

You know one thing? We humans respond to our negative feelings like they are bad, and we have trained our brains to be scared of them. To build a strong relationship with your emotions, you have to acknowledge them (whether good or bad) rather than trying to fix them.

One way of acknowledging your emotions is to label them clearly. Instead of accepting that you're feeling bad, why don't you ask yourself how you feel? Don't group your feelings into just bad and good. Try to be specific with your emotions. At a time, you can be feeling a variety of emotions. Try to differentiate every one of them; this is a major step to building a relationship with your emotions.

After mastering these emotional fitness techniques, you have to keep up with them. Try to be in the present and be aware at all times. Keep a good relationship with your emotions. Keep healthy connections and relationships. If you truly master all these, your emotions and feelings can no longer overwhelm you. Don't think being emotionally fit has nothing to do with losing weight because it has everything to do with it! Staying emotionally fit will help you achieve your goals effectively, which is to lose weight.

Creating a Personalized Weight Loss Plan

After perfecting the acts of connecting your mind and body and understanding the theory of the Law of Attraction, your body and mind will be set on losing weight. Your mind will be without doubts that you can get that body that you want, and your body will be ready to do all the work it should do to achieve that look.

At this point, you will be mentally prepared to lose weight, and the next step is the psychical work. This is why you need to create a weight loss plan. One that will fit your daily schedule and lifestyle, not just one that you find on the internet. A weight loss plan should be personalized because it is *you that want to lose weight, so you have to create *your plan. Don't you worry, in this chapter; I'll be telling you all I know about creating a weight loss plan?

The Big 5

These are the five questions you need to ask yourself before going ahead to create your weight loss plan.

1. *What time do you wake up and what time do you sleep?*

Knowing this will help you know what time to allocate your snacks and meals. If you wake up by 11 am, you can't set breakfast for 9 am, or can you? So, it is necessary to know this so that you can distribute your meals throughout the day and avoid binge eating.

2. *Eat out, how often?*

If you eat out a lot, you need to be able to account for the restaurants' meals. Find out how many calories the foods contain before eating them and if you have a special, ensure it is something healthy. This may be difficult because it won't be easy to keep track of the meals' calorie count as you're not preparing them or portioning them yourself. However, some restaurants have the calorie count of their meals displayed on their menus. Check this out before including the meals in your meal plan.

3. Emotional eater?
We've talked about emotional eating before, so I'm sure you know what it is. So, are you an emotional eater? It is very important to know this because it

can seriously affect your weight loss plan. An emotional eater eats when stressed, sad, or anxious. If you do this, you can't follow your weight loss plan. One way to help you through this is to keep a food diary where you write down your reasons or triggers for emotional eating. With this, you will be able to identify when you're triggered to eat to lift your mood, and instead of eating, try to do something else (that doesn't involve food). Let this activity you choose (maybe listening to music) replace emotional eating.

4. Do you know your food portions? Do you eat once, twice, or five times a day? How much food do you eat? You need to have the

answers to these questions. If you have many meals to pick from, it will be confusing to know how much to eat. Do not be like many people who use fullness to measure portions. If you eat till you're filled, you're going to be eating a lot! You should eat small portions of food five times a day than overfeeding yourself twice a day. So, determine your eating schedule, share your calories accordingly, and learn how to be satisfied with little food portions.

5. How much exercise can you do? To create an achievable goal, you have to be realistic. If you can't lift weights, don't put them in your weight loss plan! How much exercise can you do? How much

exercise can you devote to doing? It is recommended to do at least 30 minutes of physical activity a day, either walking or jogging. You can ask your doctor what is best for you, especially if you have health challenges.

Factors Affecting Your Weight Loss Plan

After asking yourself these questions and answering them, note these three factors that can affect what and what not to include in your weight loss plan- nutrition, exercise, and lifestyle. After fully understanding how these three factors affect your plan, you can easily go ahead and create one.

Nutrition

I'm simply going to talk about calories. Some foods have more calories than the others; fatty and sugary foods have more calories. Eat lesser calories than your body uses because if you do the opposite, your body will store them as fat. Did you know one pound of fat equals 3,500 calories? So before you can lose one pound, you have to get 3,500 calories out of your body! One way to go about this faster is to take out soda from your diet; this will remove about 350 calories a day. Some simple things you should know about dieting are:

- *Before taking "more" food, wait for 15 minutes to*

determine if you're hungry or not.

- *Eat only when you're hungry. You may eat four or five times a day but eat only when you're hungry.*

- *Eat a variety of foods. Eat veggies and fruits and whole grains. Don't eat the same thing every day.*
- *Do not skip meals; you won't lose weight that way. Instead, it might make you overeat later.*
- *Avoid packaged, fatty or sugary foods.*
- *Drink a lot of water!*

Lifestyle

You have to either make a plan that fits into your schedule or be ready to change your schedule for your plan to be successful. This could be waking up earlier than usual to go for a run before work. It could mean waking up earlier to cook so you won't have to eat out. It could mean saying goodbye to your favorite restaurant. You may have to add more hours to your sleeping time because enough sleep can help with weight loss. You may have to reduce your stress level by figuring out what stresses you out and avoiding them. What I'm saying, in essence, is that your weight loss plan must blend into your lifestyle.

Exercise
Even if you aren't trying to lose weight, exercising should be a part of your daily schedule. Why? Because it keeps you in good health. Everyone should get regular physical activity, whether overweight or slim, young or old. Here are some

simple physical activities you can engage in:

- *Do household chores like weeding or vacuuming.*
- *Add ten minutes more to your exercise time.*
- *Park further from your destination and walk. Or walk from home instead, if possible.*
- *Instead of elevators, take the stairs.*
- *Go for hikes or bike rides.*
- *Limit the time you spend with your phone or watching TV.*
- *Go for a run with pets, family, or friends.*
- *You can challenge yourself! Do something more intense than what you do now!*

Creating Your Plan

Now you have considered all the factors involved in making your weight loss plan;

what comes next is making the plan. Here is a list of what your plan should be all about;

Know your weight and BMI

To calculate your BMI (Body Mass Index), you can use a BMI calculator. Enter your height and weight into the calculator, and it will display your BMI. Doctors use BMI to measure health risk as terms like obesity and overweight are based on the BMI scale. The higher your BMI is, the greater your risk of having a weight-related illness is.

Set achievable goals. If you want to lose weight, set goals that are possible to achieve. Don't expect to lose 60 pounds before the reunion next week! That's impossible! Instead, commit to losing at least two pounds per week. This way, you go slow, dedicated, and steady, and before you know it, you're shedding weight.

Create an exercise routine

I have already listed a couple of physical activities you could do. So, you can incorporate some of them into your plan. However, try to incorporate some intense exercise as well so that you break more sweat and lose more weight. Note that whatever exercises you choose to engage in, you must do them happily and not like you're compelled to do them.

Create a diet plan

If you're a very busy person, it

may be difficult to follow this plan,
I know. But, if you want this to
work out, you must stick to this
plan. Clear out the junk foods in
your refrigerator and put in
veggies, fruits, fresh foods, and
lean proteins. I'll talk more about
such foods in the next chapter.

Keep track of your progress.

Apart from writing affirmations
down, you should keep a fitness
journal to keep track of your
progress. You write down what
you're eating and what you're not.
You write how well you're
following your exercise routines.
You know, keep tabs on yourself,
and as you review them, you get to
know if the plan is working for
you and how close to success you
are.

These are everything you need to
know about creating a weight loss

plan. Immediately after reading this book, I want you to go ahead and create your weight loss plan. In the next two chapters, I'll give you healthy foods and drinks to help you create your diet plan.

You might consult your doctor or dietician to assist you and you can make it yourself. But I want you to promise me you're going to make one. Why is it necessary? It is because it's going to be your guide throughout your journey, and it's going to keep you in check. I wouldn't be telling you to create one if it hadn't worked for me so, go ahead and create yours!

Weight Loss Recipes: Foods

Because I care about you and have promised to provide you with as much help as I can for your weight loss journey, I'll be giving you, in this chapter, some recipes you can include in your meal or diet plan. Generally, foods like whole eggs, boiled potatoes, soups, and salmon are great for weight loss. However, in this chapter, I'll give you a list of meals you can easily prepare by yourself for either breakfast, lunch, or dinner. I'd have loved to share the cooking procedures with you, but I don't know so much about cooking, I must *confess. You can easily get some food ideas from here and check out how to prepare them on the internet. I hope you're okay with that.*

Why You Need to Plan Your Meals

Before I go on to list the foods, I'd like to share with you the reasons why having a meal plan is essential. Your meal plan falls under your weight loss plan, and the latter can't be complete without a meal plan. This plan may be made weekly or monthly because changing the meals on the list will add variety and fun to it. The plan should include your breakfast, lunch, and dinner for each day and what time you eat them. Here are the reasons you need a meal/diet plan;

- *It saves time*

Thinking about what to prepare every day takes a lot of time. You spend a lot of time grocery shopping and cleaning up after meals, and you don't need to waste more time thinking of what to cook. By planning your meals for the week, you focus on shopping for groceries, and you prevent overspending when you are there.

- *It prevents unhealthy options.* When you have a food plan, you avoid last-minute orders or takeaways. Most of these meals are unhealthy and contain a lot of calories. Most people opt for these meals when they're tired or stressed, and being hungry and tired leads to unhealthy food choices. But, when there's already a plan, you know what to cook, and all you have to do is cook it.

- It controls portions and avoids waste.

With a meal plan, you avoid overeating as you already have your portions planned. And when you prepare your right portion of food, there won't be any leftover to waste.

- It allows a variety

It is very easy to eat the same thing over and again when you're a busy person. But your meal plan allows you to include a variety of foods, including vegetables and fruits. This helps you make healthier choices of food.

Now that you understand the benefits of creating a meal plan, here are a variety of weight-loss foods you can include in your plan for breakfast, lunch, or dinner. Let's categorize them first.

> Low carbohydrate foods
These are foods that contain fewer carbs but provide us with the required energy to get through the day.
Meat — Beef, Chicken, Turkey Lamb, Jerky, and Eggs Seafood — Salmon, Sardines, Trout, Lobster, and Catfish

> Low carbs vegetables
Vegetables are typically low in carbs. However, we will go for the ones that are nutrient -packed and ensure you feel and look healthy. At the same time, they don't contribute to weight loss.
Less than 5% of carbs per 100grams — Tomatoes, Cucumber, Asparagus, and Mushrooms

5%-10% of carbs per 100grams —
Cauliflower, Broccoli, Onion,
Eggplant, Green Beans, Bell
Peppers.

> *Fibrous Rich foods*
Consuming foods high in fiber
prompt weight loss by controlling
our food portions, especially of
dense carbohydrate foods.
All the vegetables previously
listed are rich in fiber, but some
foods contain more. Fibrous
rich foods — Avocados,
Almonds, Chia Seeds (one of the
highest), Peanuts, and Kale.

> *Healthy fatty foods*
We need healthy fats to work off
body fat in the body at the same
time, complementing our diet.

Here are some foods that contain healthy fats.
Extra Virgin Olive Oil, Cheese, Dark Chocolate, and Coconut Oil.

> Fruits

Fruits are sources of both minerals and vitamins. They do not directly help you lose weight. However, vitamins and minerals ensure your body is aptly functioning for weight loss. Simply, these nutrients ensure you stay healthy while you burn fat. Here are some of them.

Apricot, Blueberries,

Strawberries,

Grapefruits, and Olives.

Some outcomes:

1. Blueberry Lemon Ricotta Pancakes
No better way to begin the list than with delicious pancakes. These pancakes contain just 310 calories and are made with yogurt and cottage cheese; these give you extra protein and are the lightest pancakes you've ever had. For this meal (which is best as breakfast), you will need blueberries (of course!), sugar, water, lemon, yogurt...and a few other ingredients.

2. Chicken Fried Rice
The name of the meal already sounds delicious! You see that weight loss meals don't just include veggies. This meal

contains about 390 calories and is nutritious for you; I mean, we're talking about white rice here. That's one of the most nutritious staples ever. You'll need some carrots, rice, eggs, and a couple of other things, oh yes, skinless chicken thighs!

3. Butternut Squash Soup
If you're not a soup lover, you better get yourself to be one. Why? Because soups are fantastic for losing weight. This soup, the butternut squash, contains 150 calories and is the first I'm talking about today because it'll get you licking your lips. It is really tasty, and again, it is very healthy and packed up with many vitamins. Ingredients used to

prepare this soup include butternut squash, nutmeg, bacon, and ginger.

4. Spicy Tomato Sauce Spaghetti and Bacon

Are you surprised I'm not writing stuff like apple slices and bowls of veggies? Well, when trying to lose weight, you can eat food so long as it's healthy and nutritious for you. Just watch your portions! Now, I'm a sucker for spaghetti, which is one of my favorites on the list. You don't even need beef for this meal because the bacon does all the "meaty" work and gives it a rich and spicy taste. In total, the meal contains 370 calories, and you'll need bacon, tomatoes, spaghetti, and to give it that hot taste, pepper flakes.

5. Caribbean Steamed Fish
Herbs and spices are extraordinary with the way they can change something bland to a delicious meal. This meal, for example, is fish. The fish comes out tasting like the most flavored and spiciest thing on earth with the spices and herbs it is garnished with. For this dramatic transformation (from bland to spicy), you need ingredients like lime, carrots, hot pepper, butter, and okra.

6. Tuna Poke Bowls
With tuna, mayonnaise, sriracha, cucumbers, white rice,

*scallions, and avocado, you can
prepare yourself a nutritious
plate of spicy tuna poke bowls
for breakfast. The meal contains
various healthy ingredients like
cucumbers, which are low in
calories and are beneficial for
weight loss (of course), digestive
regularity, and lowering blood
sugar levels.*

7. Oatmeal Pancakes with Cinnamon
   Apples

*This is another interesting and
nutritious meal I love. The wheat
flour and oats give the pancakes
a protein and fiber boost that
stabilizes blood sugar levels.
The meal contains 260 calories,
and you'll need wheat flour,
oats, baking powder, cinnamon,*

buttermilk, brown sugar, and apples to do the magic.

8. Avocado Salad and Grilled Chicken

We finally get to talk about salad. You should know that your salad should be made by

you and nobody else. Salads are great because they are good for you (obviously) and are filled with nutritious ingredients. This Avocado salad is rich in protein, contains 500 calories, and is great for weight loss. All you need for this salad are chicken, goat cheese, arugula, avocado, walnuts, dried cranberries, and honey mustard vinaigrette.

Are You a Vegetarian?
If your answer's yes, don't you worry, I've got you covered. I'll give you a list of meat-free meals that aren't the pasta and veggies you may be used to.

1. French Toast Stuffed with Strawberries

Hearing the word "stuffed", you are probably thinking the sandwich is filled with unhealthy ingredients that contain fat, salt, and sugar. Well, that's not the case here. The stuffing in this sandwich contains fiber, protein, and vitamins. This meal can easily be pulled off as breakfast, and you'll need ingredients like cottage cheese, eggs, cinnamon, whole wheat bread, and strawberries. This meal is so delicious you wouldn't think it's healthy.

2. Banana Pancakes

These pancakes contain 320 calories and are most likely the lightest and moistest pancakes you'll ever eat. The cottage cheese and yogurt give the extra meal protein, and the fresh banana slices turn golden brown once they hit the skillet. To make this meal, you need yogurt, lemon juice, cottage cheese, sliced bananas, and baking soda.

3. Pickled Cucumber Salad

Do you know why I love salads? It's because most of the time, you don't have to cook anything up! You just throw in veggies and fruits, and ta-dah, your meal is ready. This meal can be used as a condiment or side dish. The salad can be served with almost everything- chicken, steak, or salmon (oh, you're vegan, I forgot!). The cucumber salad can be kept in the refrigerator for five days, at least, and can be a go-to meal for those busy nights. Like I said already, you don't have to cook anything, just throw in your sliced cucumber, sliced onions, and other ingredients into a bowl, mix them up, wait for a while, and your salad is ready.

4. Shakshuka

This is a North African dish made of pepper sauce and eggs poached in garlicky tomato. To make the dish, you need fresh or canned tomatoes, peppers, garlic, and onion. To bring out the spicy taste and to make the shakshuka more exciting than the everyday tomato and garlic sauce, add a spoonful of the Northern American red pepper.

5. Gazpacho

Instead of the basic tomato soup, why don't you try out gazpacho, which is like a garden in a bowl? Gazpacho is preferable to ordinary tomato soup because it's more complex and contains more flavors and greenery. Containing just 120 calories, the gazpacho is instantly going to become one of your favorites once it touches your tongue.

I hope you can pick at least five meals from the list to add to your meal plan. Remember, you need a variety of meals and not a repetition. If this list isn't satisfactory for you, go ahead and ask your doctor or dietician or the internet. I care about your well -being and journey, so; I want you to do everything you can to lose that weight. This chapter's main point is to get you to create a meal plan containing a variety of meals; now, get to it!

Weight Loss Recipes: Drinks

Apart from foods, certain drinks support weight loss and should also be added to your diet plan. These drinks help you keep away hunger pangs that make you overeat or eat unhealthy foods. They also increase your metabolism and aid your weight loss efforts. I'll share some common drinks with you and some that I specifically used during my weight loss journey.

Common Weight Loss Drinks

We take some of these drinks daily and don't even know they are beneficial for weight loss. They increase metabolism and fullness, which both result in weight loss.

These drinks include water, coffee, green tea, and apple cider vinegar drinks.

Water

Drinking enough water each day is one of the easiest ways to improve your general health.

Water:

increases the number of calories you burn, and this is known as resting energy expenditure. This result will be more impressive when the water is cold because the body uses extra calories to warm the water to the normal body temperature.

When drunk before meals, it reduces the appetite in older and middle-aged individuals, thereby preventing overeating.

Intake for a day should be 1 to 2 liters to assist with weight loss.

Coffee

Coffee is another drink that propagates weight loss. Many of us don't know this, and we just drink coffee for the sake of it. Well, if you want to be intentional about it for weight loss, it involves drinking a minimum of 3 cups of light-roast coffee every day. It is healthier to prepare your coffee at home by grinding lightly roasted, whole-bean coffee and preparing with filtered water. Some benefits of coffee are:

- *It suppresses appetite (drinking coffee before eating will decrease how much you eat), and this decreases your calorie intake.*

- *It increases metabolism.*
- *It increases the amount of fat you burn during a workout.*

Green Tea

Green tea has been proven to be one of the most effective drinks for weight loss. Drinking the tea decreases body weight and fat, just like the other drinks on the list. This benefit results from the antioxidants used in the tea preparation, which burns fat and increases metabolism.

It also contains caffeine, which boosts energy levels and improves performance when exercising. Drinking 2-3 cups a day helps in supplementing weight loss.

Apple Cider Vinegar Drinks

This is one drink you need to consult a specialist before going ahead to add it to your meal plan. This is because there are some consequences when you take too much of it. On the other hand, the drink:

- *Decreases insulin levels and burns fat.*
- *Keeps you full for a long time as it slows the emptying of the stomach.*
- *Stabilizes blood sugar, especially after eating a meal that is high in carbohydrates.*

Drinks That Worked for Me

I mentioned earlier that I would share with you drinks that I used during my journey, which worked for me. These drinks include water and lemon, lemon and ginger tea, and Super Greens. I added them to my plan, and alongside healthy foods, regular exercise, and the successful connection of my body and mind, I was able to lose weight. By incorporating these drinks into your plan, you are most likely to get the results I got. Let's begin, shall we?

Water and Lemon
Water and lemon are commonly referred to as lemon water. It is a beverage made by mixing water and fresh lemon juice, which can be enjoyed either hot or cold. The drink is said to have many

benefits, such as increasing energy levels and improving digestion. However, the benefit we are focused on is the benefit of promoting weight loss. How does it do that? Well, I'll tell you below;

> It keeps you hydrated. Lemon water is majorly made up of water, and water keeps the body hydrated. Staying hydrated is a critical component of health and is essential for regulating body temperature and improving its physical performance. Also, staying hydrated aids weight loss as research has shown that an increase in hydration leads to an increase in fats' breakdown in

the body. It also prevents
bloating and weight gain by
reducing water retention.

> It is very low in calories.
Replacing drinks like orange
juice or soda for lemon water is a
safe and healthy choice because
of the few calories it contains
compared to the other two
drinks. For example, if you
squeeze out the juice from half a
lemon into water, a glass of the
lemon water will contain just 6
calories. A cup of orange juice
contains 110 calories. Can you
see the difference? So, drinking
lemon water instead of the other
drinks your calorie intake by

about 100 calories.

> It boosts metabolism
*Drinking lemon water has similar
advantages to drinking enough
water, and this is because the
drink majorly contains water. So,
drinking lemon water, just like
drinking water, enhances
mitochondria's function (which
generates energy for the body),
which increases metabolism. This,
in the long run, leads to weight
loss.*

Lemon and Ginger Tea
*This is another natural, herbal,
and homemade drink that helped
me achieve my weight loss goals.
If you haven't noticed, all the
drinks I've listed so far are*

natural, and you can easily make them yourself. This way, you can be sure of what you're drinking and be completely sure it's 100% nutritious and 0% harmful.

Making the lemon and ginger tea is quite easy; all you need are lemon juice, grated ginger, and honey. Mix all the ingredients in a bowl and then keep them overnight in the refrigerator. By the next morning, the mixture will be thick; and to make your tea, add a teaspoon of the mixture into a cup of water, and ta-dah, your lemon and ginger tea is ready! Here are some benefits of this tea;

> It reduces oxidative stress.

If you can remember, we talked about the effect of stress on your eating habits some chapters ago. Ginger, which is a major ingredient in the tea, aids pain relief, including stress and headaches. It contains an antioxidant gingerol, which fights chemicals of your body that cause physical and psychological stress. By reducing stress, the tea reduces your chances of emotional eating.

> *It aids digestion and stabilizes blood sugar levels.*

Ginger increases your "digestive fire" and helps you break down your food easily. It eliminates gas from the body and relaxes the intestines' muscles. This quality of the drink assists in the weight loss process.

> *It is a filling drink.*

The ginger and lemon tea acts as an appetite suppressant and stops you from eating unnecessarily (binge eating). By drinking more of this tea, you are less likely to get hungry as much as you were when you weren't drinking it. In summary, this drink helps you feel fuller for a longer time, thereby preventing you from overeating.

> Super Greens

Now, this is a product I can proudly say worked for me. I'm excited to be sharing it with you because I'm sure it's going to help you as it did me!

Super Greens are simply made of dried dietary supplements that you can mix with water or other liquids. Generally, Super Greens have about 30 different *ingredients, and some of them are grasses, green vegetables, extra fiber, high-antioxidant fruits, and digestive enzymes. The Super Greens product I use contains barley grass, broccoli powder, wheatgrass, spinach powder, apple powder, and beetroot powder, among many others.*

I drink my Super Greens in the morning after breakfast, and it gives me energy that lasts throughout the whole day! Some people prefer to take first thing in the morning, even before breakfast. But generally, taking your Super Greens in the morning fills your body system with nutrients and gives your day a good start. This doesn't mean it can't be beneficial at another time of the day. So that you know, it is an ideal energy booster in the afternoon too!

What to mix your Super Greens with? You can mix it with just about anything! I mix mine with milk, but there are so many other options. Most people mix theirs in water and some in their smoothie or juice. It blends easily into whatever you're mixing it with, but that doesn't mean its nutrients are silenced. Here are the benefits of this Super Greens *that make me love it so much;*

> *It helps to eliminate cravings.*
*Although Super Greens have not
been proven to help with weight
loss, it does a great job of
eliminating cravings and
suppressing the appetite.
Because of the many nutrients it
provides to the body, your
hypothalamus stops sending
hunger signals to the brain.
Fewer cravings lead to less
appetite, which leads to fewer
calories, which leads to weight
loss!*

> *It gives energy*
*This is why I love it so much and
still drink it to date. It promotes*

the energy level without the crash you get from other substances like sugar, energy drinks, or caffeine. It enables focus and clear thinking, and that's why it is best to take it at the start of the day.

> *It aids digestion and prevents bloating.*

Your gut struggles to deal with healthy and bad foods you eat when your digestive system is compromised. The digestive enzymes included in the Super Greens your guts to extract maximum nutrients from it and every other meal on your diet. The enzymes allow your gut to handle the situations better, thereby reducing bloating or even eliminating them.

I hope that you check these drinks out and try to incorporate them into your meal plan. When you consume these drinks, do not expect to lose weight instantly. It takes patience and some time before you start seeing their effects. Just make sure to be persistent with them and the foods also and remember always to be positive. Do not forget all I've talked about from the start, and instead of seeing losing weight as an impossible task, open your mind to positivity and let the law of attraction do its work.

Conclusion

We have come to the end of this journey. Weight loss is not only a controversial concept but a very popular one. Blame the dopamine release and, consequently, its effects associated with eating. However, since we are all peculiar in our way, it poses a threat to losing weight using any of the diet plans listed.

This is why I didn't set out to teach about diet plans but how you can create your own unique weight loss program that fits perfectly with your lifestyle.

Besides creating a personalized plan, this book's intent was how your minds could either positively or negatively impact this plan. We read how to steer our minds to transform our weight loss plan positively.

Each of these concepts, the law of attraction, meditation, visualization, affirmations, and scripting, detailed how losing weight is not only about what you choose to eat or how you choose to exercise. That's all most of us can relate to weight loss and why some people still end up failing to lose weight. The mind might as well dictate our existence, as it encompasses our brain, thoughts, and psychological drive towards action. We might as well take advantage of it to shed those extra pounds.

My hope is that you do not just read the content of this book but set out to digest and implement all the ideas and see how it helps you lose weight effortlessly.

9 781801 572156